NED OVEREND

MOUNTAIN BIKE
LIKE A CHAMPION

NED OVEREND

MOUNTAIN BIKE
LIKE A CHAMPION

Master the Techniques of America's Greatest Rider

By **Ned Overend** with Ed Pavelka

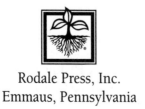

Rodale Press, Inc.
Emmaus, Pennsylvania

Notice

The information in this book is meant to supplement, not replace, proper mountain biking training. Like any sport involving speed, equipment, balance, and environmental factors, mountain biking poses some inherent risk. The authors and publisher advise readers to take full responsibility for their safety and know their limits. Before practicing the skills described in this book, be sure that your equipment is well-maintained, and do not take risks beyond your level of experience, aptitude, training, and comfort level.

Cover Design by Patrick Maley
Cover Photograph by Steve Giberson
Interior Design by Christopher Rhoads
Interior Photographs by Pam Overend, except: Simon Cudby, p. 1; Jim DeFrisco/Rodale Images, p. 63; Steve Giberson, pp. 52, 90, 103, 110, 111, 112; John P. Hamel/Rodale Images, pp. x, 151

Library of Congress Cataloging-in-Publication Data

Overend, Ned.
    Mountain bike like a champion : master the techniques of America's greatest
rider / by Ned Overend with Ed Pavelka.
        p.   cm.
    At head of title: Ned Overend
    Includes index.
    ISBN 1-57954-081-3   paperback
    1. All terrain cycling.   2. All terrain cycling—Training.   I. Pavelka, Ed.   II. Title.
III. Title: Ned Overend
GV1056.O84   1999
796.6'3—dc21   99-28633

Distributed to the book trade by St. Martin's Press

    4   6   8   10   9   7   5   paperback

Visit us on the Web at www.rodalesportsandfitness.com, or call us toll-free at (800) 848-4735.

┌─────────── OUR PURPOSE ───────────┐

*We inspire and enable people to improve
their lives and the world around them.*

└───────────────────────────────────┘

To my family,
Pam, Allison, and Rhyler

Contents

Part Three: Competition

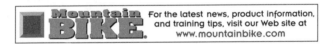
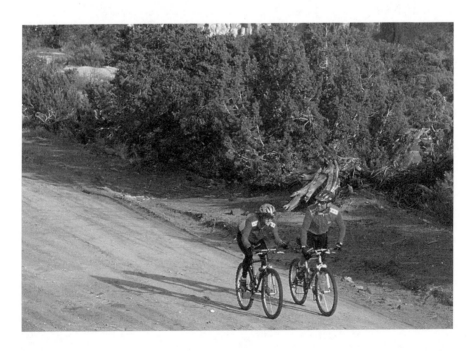

Introduction

Even 20 years ago, the first time I met Ned Overend, he stood out as a bike racer. Back then, however, it wasn't because of some sensational victory. In fact, few in cycling even knew his name, and we certainly couldn't imagine the impact he'd have on the sport. At that time, you could still count the number of mountain bikes in the entire world on your fingers. Ned's vehicle to greatness was just being born.

My recollection is of Ned competing in the Coors Classic, then America's biggest road stage race. And the reason I remember him is because he was wearing a hard-shell cycling helmet—the only one in the sea of traditional leather-strap "hairnets." It was an odd sight that caused a few disparaging comments from the purists. But Ned wasn't fazed. He was just ahead of his time. And that's the way it's been for his entire groundbreaking career.

As an athlete, Ned had it from the beginning. He ran track and cross-country in high school and college, developing a big aerobic base. He tried some new, off-beat events called triathlons while attending San Diego State University, which introduced him to cycling and eventually road racing. His move to Durango, Colorado, put him in a perfect place to get on a mountain bike when they became available in the early 1980s. The rest, as they say, is history. Ned went on to win dozens of elite off-road races, including six national championships in a seven-year stretch, plus the first official cross-country world championship in 1990. No American mountain biker can lay claim to a more successful career.

This book tells you how to ride like Ned. It covers the gamut of off-road riding techniques and equipment setup, often illustrated by war stories from races he's competed in around the world. Ned and I worked together through many weeks (and a few rides) to capture all of his knowledge, insights, and advice. His renowned good nature made our time together a pleasure. (If you get a chance to meet Ned, don't be shy. They don't call him

Mr. Nice Guy for nothing. He'll always take a moment to chat and answer your questions.) Finally, after covering dozens of essential skills, we added a special section about cross-country training and racing. If you want to compete like a champion, you now have the advantage of Ned's unparalleled knowledge.

And he's far from finished. Now in his forties, Ned has stepped back from full-time professional mountain bike racing but not from world-class competition. In 1998, he won the biggest event in an extreme sport known as X-Terra. This off-road triathlon combines open-water swimming, trail running, and, of course, mountain biking. Guess where Ned really gains ground. Here's hoping this book helps lower the other competitors' handicaps.

One note before we begin: Throughout the book, we use the masculine gender to spare readers from the unwieldy sentences that would result from joint inclusion of the masculine and feminine genders. We do this with full recognition that many of the most talented and accomplished mountain bikers are women. If this style upsets anyone, tell him/her (see?) to go for a ride to unwind. Better yet, let's all go.

Ed Pavelka

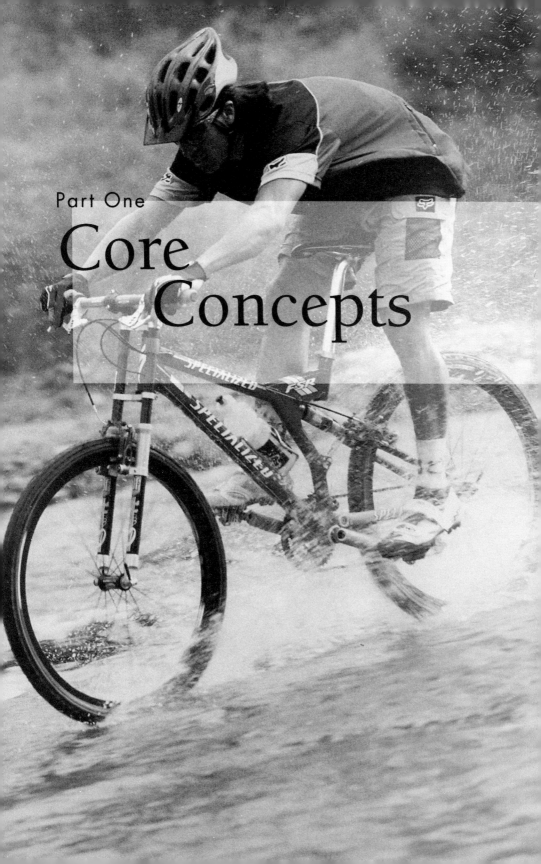

Part One

Core
Concepts

1 Riding Position

11 Steps to an Excellent Bike Fit

Roadies are known for refining their positions down to the millimeter. Mountain bikers tend to approach things more casually. At least I did, until just before a race a few seasons ago. I'd just built a new bike, and all I had on hand was a long 14.5-centimeter (cm) stem. Hey, it felt fine while I was riding around my driveway.

Unfortunately, the race was another story. When I tried to push myself back on steep descents, I couldn't. It was impossible to get enough weight off the front wheel, and as a result, I crashed several times. I was out of control.

The lesson? Establish your riding position carefully, then stick to the numbers. This is the first step in becoming the best mountain biker you can be. The main exception is if you are a young rider who occasionally needs to adjust for a growing body. Otherwise, you can set your position and forget it—unless there is a good reason to experiment, such as an injury or change in equipment.

If you decide to make a modification, do it in small increments and test the new position in all kinds of terrains and situations. Get one thing right before moving to the next. If you make multiple changes all at once, you won't be sure what is working and what isn't.

I know riders who make themselves crazy trying to find the perfect position. It probably doesn't exist. A change in handlebar height, for example, can

3

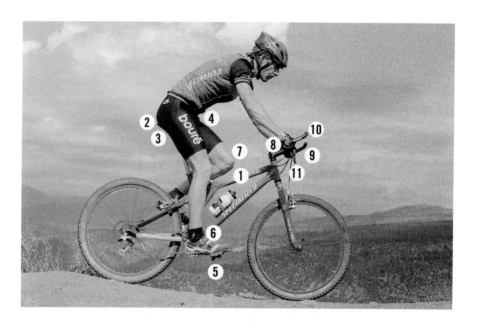

feel a little awkward at first. Don't worry about it; just get used to it once you're confident that you're within the guidelines that I'm about to give. Realize that you won't feel perfect all the time on every ride, so resist the temptation to constantly tinker. Be certain of specific needs before you make a change.

1. Frame size. As you're shopping for a bike, you need to make sure that the frame size is right. In case of spontaneous (and potentially painful) dismounts, there should be at least two inches of clearance between your crotch and the top tube. I prefer four inches, which also gives me a lighter and more compact frame.

To measure, wear your cycling shoes and stand with the bike be-tween your legs. Bikes with sloping top tubes may create even more clearance. For these, make sure that you can raise the saddle to the cor-rect height without exceeding the maximum-extension line on the seat-post when you perform step 2. You'll find this line engraved a couple of inches from the end of the post. You must also be able to achieve the proper reach (see step 7).

2. Saddle height. You'll need these props: a book, pencil, metric tape mea-sure, and calculator. It also helps to have an assistant, so invite a friend over with his bike and you can both dial your positions.

First, measure your inseam. Stand with your bare feet about six inches apart facing a wall. Place the book between your legs with one edge flat to the wall, then slide it up until it's snug in your crotch. Mark the wall at the top corner of the book. Measure from the floor to the mark (your in-seam length), then multiply this number by 0.883. The result is the proper distance from the center of the crankarm axle to the top of the saddle, measured in line with the seatpost. (For me, this means 82 cm × 0.883, or a 72.4-cm saddle height.)

This formula works well for most riders, but the height may need to be increased if you wear shoes with particularly thick soles or if you have feet that are large in proportion to your height. Conversely, if your hips rock to help you reach the pedals while you're riding, lower the saddle. At the bottom of the stroke, you should still have enough bend in your knees to let them absorb shock. For most riders, this means an angle of 150 to 160 degrees behind the knee when the crankarm is in line with the seat tube and the pedal is parallel to the ground.

3. Fore/aft saddle position. First, a rule: Don't move the saddle backward or forward to compensate for improper reach (the combined length of the top tube and stem). Instead, the fore/aft saddle adjust-

Tech Tip

Many experienced riders can describe at least one harrowing crash that split their helmets instead of their skulls. The story always ends with, "I wouldn't be here today if I hadn't been wearing that thing." But to get a helmet's full protection, you have to adjust it properly. Many riders don't.

The problem I often see is a loose fit. Assuming that the helmet is the correct basic size for your head, use the supplied pads to make it fit snugly without any uncomfortable pressure spots. It should sit squarely on your head, about a finger's width up from your eyebrows. Buckle up, then grasp the helmet with both hands and try to move it from side to side and from front to back. If moderate force causes it to slip by more than an inch, tighten the strap. You need to approach the point where you start to feel the strap pressing your throat when you swallow. Be sure to hold your head and neck in the same position as when riding.

Some helmets come with a retention system that cradles the lower rear portion of your head. This is the type you want for mountain biking. It creates a more secure fit that stops the helmet from rattling on a rough trail or dislodging when you go cartwheeling in a crash. Half of your clothes may fly off, but your helmet must stay on.

ment is for establishing your position relative to the pedals. Put your bike on an indoor trainer or next to a wall. Climb on, wearing your cycling shoes. Sit normally in the center of the saddle. Clip into the pedals and position the crankarms horizontally. Have your friend drop a plumb line (a string with something small but heavy on the end) from the front of your forward leg's kneecap. The string should touch the end of the crankarm. This is the neutral, or 0, position, which works well for most riders.

However, if you like to push bigger gears with a slower cadence, a knee position up to 6 cm behind 0 will give you extra leverage. If you prefer spinning lower gears with a faster cadence, you'll do better at 0. Adjust the saddle accordingly. When riding, you can change this relationship simply by sliding on the saddle, moving in front of 0 or behind 0, depending on the conditions. My basic position is about 4 cm behind 0. This allows me to slide forward over the pedals for steep climbing or slide backward to gain more leg extension for power on the flats.

4. Saddle tilt. Lay a yardstick along the length of the saddle to see its angle. Do this with the bike on a level surface (like the floor) with something horizontal in the background (like a windowsill) to compare to the yardstick. A level saddle works well for the road, but for mountain biking, I recommend tipping the nose down a degree or two. Be careful. A little downward tilt can reduce crotch pressure and make it easier to move back and forth, but too much will cause you to constantly slide forward and put excessive weight on your arms. Never

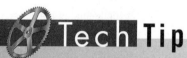

Tech Tip

Okay, you've carefully worked your way through all of your riding-position checks. You've ridden in a range of situations to test how well your position works. You've tweaked a couple of things. You have it nailed. Think you're done? Not quite.

There's one final step. You need to carefully record all of the measurements and keep them in your training log, toolbox, or another safe place. Then, if you crash and knock things out of place or need to install new parts, you'll know exactly how to position them. You'll also have a much easier time setting up a loaner bike or even your next new one.

Remember, your ideal position results from adjusting your bike to fit your body, not forcing your body to accommodate the bike.

angle the nose up. It will press harder into your crotch and snag your shorts when you go from standing to sitting.

5. Foot position on the pedal. Adjust each cleat fore and aft to put the ball of your foot directly over or as much as 5 millimeters (mm) in front of the pedal axle. (If the ball is behind the axle, you'll pedal on your toes and risk straining the muscles and tendons of your foot and calf.) I recommend clipless pedals that allow your feet to pivot, or float, a few degrees before releasing. This lets your feet assume their natural angles on the pedals. Your ankles and knees will thank you. Adjust the cleat angle so your heel has to travel the same distance left or right to reach the release point. Check this with your bike on a stationary trainer. Pedal easily to let your feet find their natural positions, then repeatedly release to the inside and outside. Keep adjusting until you have it right for both feet.

6. Crankarm length. In general, mountain bikers benefit from long levers. So for optimum pedaling power, all but the smallest riders (shorter than 5 foot 4) should use 175-mm crankarms rather than the 170-mm length commonly found on road bikes. Small-frame mountain bikes should come with 170s to make them proportionally correct for short riders. The length is stamped on the back of each crankarm.

7. Cockpit dimensions. The key requirement in the driver compartment is to have enough room to move and apply body English. When you're standing and the wheel is pointed straight ahead, make sure that there is at least an inch of clearance between the handlebar grips and your knees when they're fully to the front. This lets you pedal while surging forward to get your wheel over an obstacle. My setup gives me 2 inches, a margin that's especially helpful in the woods when the handlebar is being worked hard to steer through tight places. If your knees come too close or even hit, you need more reach. Hopefully, you can make the correction with a longer stem and not have to swap the frame for one that has a longer top tube. Conversely, your handlebar must be close enough to let you extend your arms and push your butt all the way behind the saddle. You need this position for steep downhills and drop-offs.

8. Handlebar and stem height. Here's what to look for: When riding normally with slightly bent elbows, you should have roughly a 45-degree bend at the waist. From this position, you can lower your chest for a more aero position at high speeds and to weight the front wheel for steering traction on climbs. But you also can raise your chest to lighten the front wheel over obstacles and increase weight on the rear wheel for climbing traction.

9. Handlebar bend and width. Most flat bars have a rearward bend, or sweep, of three degrees. I like to position mine to give me the most natural angle for my wrists. If necessary, shorten your bar with a hacksaw or pipe cutter so the grips are at shoulder width (or just slightly wider), which helps you pull straight back while climbing.

Riser bars are appearing on all types of mountain bikes, not just on the downhill machines where they gained popularity. As opposed to traditional flat bars, risers have an upward bend and one to three inches more width. They give you a more upright position, help you get your weight off the front wheel so you can loft it easier, and slow your steering input slightly to increase stability. All of these things help a downhiller and they're fine for recreational trail riding, too. But I recommend flat bars for cross-country racing. Being narrower, a flat bar helps you steer more quickly and squeeze through trees and other tight places. It's also better for climbing. And whenever you reach a fast, open stretch, a flat bar helps you get lower and more aerodynamic to boost speed.

10. Bar-end position. If you use them, bar-ends should be positioned so your wrists are straight (not cocked) while you're standing. This lets you apply maximum torque on out-of-saddle climbs, which is where bar-ends are most useful.

11. Brake-lever position. You tend to squeeze the levers hardest when standing, crouched above the bike on a steep descent. This is the situation in which the levers need to be most accessible and comfortable. Rotate them so that in this riding position they give you straight (not cocked) wrists. If you set them for ideal access when you're in the saddle, your wrists will be at too sharp an angle when you stand.

2 Balance

The Starting Point for All Bike-Handling Skills

The dynamics of every technique that I discuss in this book rely on one thing: your understanding of how you interact with the bike. By this, I mean how you shift your weight and how you balance. Mastering these two things, along with learning how to pedal efficiently, creates the framework for making every key move on a mountain bike—climbing, descending, braking, turning, and negotiating varied terrain.

You can develop basic skills through experience, of course, but there's a better way. By first understanding the techniques and then practicing them with specific drills, you will speed up your improvement. Very soon, you'll have more control and confidence, and you'll anxiously look forward to adding advanced skills to your arsenal.

The Human Gyroscope

If I had to give you just one example of a rider who capitalizes on balance, it would be my good friend and fellow pro racer John Tomac. In fact, he does everything so well that you're going to see his name pop up to illustrate techniques throughout this book. He and I have battled in numerous races around the world, so I've watched him perform in many different situations. I think of him as the human gyroscope. It's incredible

9

how fast he can go down a hill without falling. I don't think anyone has a greater variety of bike-handling maneuvers.

I'll never forget a move that John made at the World Cup race in Houffalize, Belgium. It was a wet morning, with 140 guys stampeding up a paved road before cutting off into the dirt. This section immediately funneled us into a rocky, slippery, steep downhill. There were maybe five lines you could take. I was in pretty good position, about 20th place, but the descent was thick with guys everywhere.

As I was going down this greasy slope, my front wheel hit a rock and deflected me on an angle. So now I was traversing across, and I just had to go with it. Unfortunately, the guy I was veering into was John Tomac. He saw me coming out of the corner of his eye. He leaned into me, hit me with his shoulder, and pivoted me off in the other direction. Before I knew it, I was in the bushes and a hundred guys were riding past. John didn't lose an inch, thanks to his split-second reaction and great balance. If I had ridden into a less-skilled rider, I probably would have knocked him down while keeping my own place in the pack. But there I was, trying to pull my bike out of the plants while John and almost everyone else were riding away.

Balancing Act

Great riding starts with great balance. You don't just ride a bike, you interact with it. By moving your arms, shoulders, and hips, you can reposition your weight to maximize performance. Balance means working with your bike instead of just sitting on it. This is essential to maintaining traction for turning, climbing, and braking.

Riding on tricky trails with hills, turns, rocks, and a narrow track—what is called technical terrain—requires the widest range of body movements. When seated, you can move only so much. But when you stand, your range of motion increases and you get another important benefit: shock absorption through your flexed legs. Although your feet and hands are attached to the bike, your upper body is free to move around the bike. Think of a three-dimensional cone extending upward from the pedals. Your body movements are in this cone, and when you stand, you increase its size. This gives you more control over your body and, thus, over the bike.

Moving your body also allows you to shift the focal point of your weight from the saddle to the pedals to the handlebar. You can add weight to either wheel to improve traction for braking, climbing, or turning. You can also take weight off either wheel to roll over obstacles more easily. By springing

Ned's KNOWLEDGE

The more people you ride with, the more often you'll be stopped for things like flat tires, crashes, trailside snacks, or trips to the bushes. Don't just stand there impatiently waiting for your buddy to hurry up. Use these delays to practice balancing techniques.

Instead of leaning on your bike while shooting the breeze, chat from a trackstand. Rather than getting off to walk back to where your friend stopped to pull the stick from his derailleur, make a tight U-turn to practice your switchback technique. Challenge someone to a slow race. See that log 30 feet away? The last one to get there wins. You're out if you put a foot down.

Slow races are instructional as well as fun. Suddenly, you are being distracted by lots of things as you try to hold your trackstand and maintain slow-speed balance. It's great for developing concentration in addition to body control. By using unplanned stops this way, they'll be less frustrating and even beneficial.

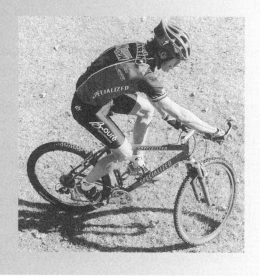

By learning to do a trackstand, you can confidently pause at any time to size up your next move. This skill hones your slow-speed balancing ability and will greatly reduce topple-over crashes.

upward, you can unweight both wheels simultaneously to fly the bike over something that you'd rather not ride into—a rock, log, ledge, ditch, or anything else just as risky.

Attack Position

When riding technical sections, assume what I call the attack position. Do this by standing in a low, balanced posture, bent at the waist. Your butt should be close to the saddle but not touching it, so your cone of move-

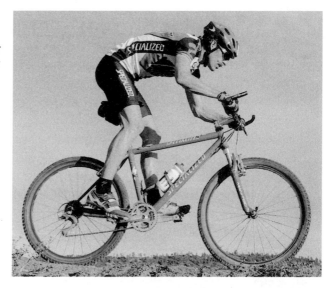

The basic attack position lets you float over rough ground. Keep your butt off the saddle, your weight centered, the crankarms horizontal, and your knees and elbows flexed to absorb shock.

ment is larger. Hold the crankarms horizontal. Flex your knees so they can soak up bumps. Keep a firm grip, but don't let your arms and shoulders become rigid. Think of your extremities as shock absorbers, protecting your torso and head from jolts. You should feel like a cat that is crouched and ready to pounce.

This position improves your ability to control the bike in tricky terrain, but it won't work without good balance. When your wheels are rolling fast, gyroscopic forces help keep the bike upright and stable. The slower you're going, the more actively you must balance the bike.

Here's a quick way to see what I mean. Remove the front wheel from your bike. Hold it upright by each end of the axle and get it spinning fast. Notice how slight the forces are when the wheel is vertical. Tilt the wheel to either side and you'll feel how it fights to get upright again. Now do the same thing with the wheel spinning much slower. Not nearly the same resistance, eh? Vertical is how a rotating wheel wants to be, but the slower it's spinning, the less help you get from gyro forces. Your ability to balance becomes much more important.

Relax

Relaxation and confidence are the two keys to balancing better. When you're relaxed, you can make precise steering adjustments to the front wheel, put traction to the rear wheel, and change your body position—all

Balance must become ingrained. You can't think about staying upright on technical trails when you need to concentrate on traction, getting over obstacles, and making tight turns. Specific practice helps. Here's how.

At a slow speed, stand, coast, and experiment with your range of motion. Work on maximizing the size of your "cone," the area that extends upward from the pedals and in which you make your body movements. Get comfortable doing this while the bike is barely rolling. Extend your body to the left, right, front, and back while maintaining a straight line with the bike. Then try it while making slow turns. Do drills like this on soft grassy areas without rocks, so if you do take a tumble, you won't get hurt. Always wear your helmet and gloves.

Learn to do a trackstand, which means to fully stop without putting a foot down. On a technical trail, a trackstand lets you pause to decide what to do next, and it may save you from toppling over if you suddenly come to an unexpected halt.

Here's how to practice trackstands. If you're confident in your ability to get out of the pedals quickly, clip in. If not, don't engage the cleats until you get the hang of this. Roll slowly to a stop with the crankarms horizontal. Try this both sitting and standing. To obtain a nearly motionless balance, squeeze the brakes, turn the wheel to one side or the other, and press against the pedals to establish equilibrium. This is a true trackstand like trackies do on a velodrome or roadies do while waiting for a traffic light. When you're good, you can remain stationary for minutes.

The alternative is to load the pedals evenly and not lock the brakes, maintaining balance by turning the front wheel from side to side, as necessary, while making slight weight shifts. You must be fairly relaxed so that your movements are subtle. If you're jerky, you'll shift your weight too far to one side. You'll tip over or need to start rolling again to regain balance.

Once you have it, graduate to uneven and varied terrain. If you're on a slope, turn the front wheel uphill and put just enough pressure on the pedals to counter the bike's tendency to roll back. This will keep you stationary.

The ultimate goal is for a trackstand to replace putting a foot down as your automatic response when something brings you to a stop. Use a trackstand to pause, size up the situation, and plan your next move.

If you're riding alone, try what I often do. On a gradual slope with good traction, ride up at a really slow speed and come to a complete stop at certain points, then move forward again. This is a great drill for coping with what happens on many climbs. Something kills your momentum and stops you dead for a split second. A lot of riders never consider continuing—they automatically put a foot down. Your instinct should be to relax, balance, point your wheel where it should go, and smoothly resume pedaling.

while concentrating on the line you want to take. During low-speed technical maneuvers, you have almost no gyro forces to help you stay upright, so your balance depends on relaxed body control.

By practicing balancing skills and trackstands, you'll develop the confidence to ride slowly. And it does take confidence. People usually think that mountain biking injuries happen only at fast speeds. Those that do certainly provide exciting videotape. But from what I've seen, most injuries actually occur when riders are going too slow to maintain balance. It's typical to fall over and get cuts and bruises or maybe even break a wrist or collarbone.

When you lose your gyro, a fall may be only an instant away—unless you've developed the right instincts. One of them is getting your feet out of the pedals and onto the ground the second you realize that tipping over is unavoidable. You'll find tips for this in chapter 3, Pedaling, and chapter 16, Switchbacks.

One place where good balance is essential is on the famous slickrock around Moab, Utah. Riding the slickrock is a must for most mountain bikers, but I'll warn you, it's very unforgiving. A couple of years ago, a guy in front of me stalled while climbing a steep pitch. This happens a lot because the transitions are so abrupt, like on a roller coaster. He was putting all of his power into the pedals and didn't have time to pull a foot out when his momentum stopped. Instead of balancing and staying in control, he fell over and tumbled back down the slope, breaking his ankle. The carnage on the slickrock is unbelievable, but a lot of it could be avoided if riders had better slow-speed control. If you can balance, you can give yourself just enough time to make an injury-preventing move.

3 Pedaling

Pedal in Circles
to Develop Efficiency and Power

Marty Nothstein may not be a mountain biker but he's still a rider whom all of us should copy. He has an unbelievably smooth and powerful pedal stroke. As a world-champion track racer, Marty needs to accelerate instantly from a cadence of around 60 rpm to more than twice as fast, using a single gear on a steeply banked velodrome. Marty is a huge guy and yet he's able to put all of this power into a sliver of a rear-tire contact patch (the section in contact with the ground) that is only a couple of centimeters long. This is just a fraction of the size of the contact patch on mountain bike tires.

When you watch Marty ride, you see a beautiful example of circular pedaling. This is what it takes to efficiently apply force through the rear wheel and smooth out the power pulses of each leg's downstrokes. In mountain biking, a circular style improves traction by reducing wheel surges and bouncing. It also helps you ride longer and stronger because it distributes the workload over a range of muscles.

To get these benefits, you need to envision pedaling as a round motion, not an up-and-down motion. Good technique consists of pushing down from the top of the stroke, dragging your foot across the bottom, then driving your knee toward the handlebar. The objective is called pedaling in circles, but in reality it's hard to concentrate on this when your legs are spinning quickly and your attention is on where your wheels are going next.

15

Rather than think about circles, make them occur automatically by mastering these four components.

1. Downstroke. This is a natural action. Everyone who rides a bike can push the pedals down using their quadriceps, which are in the front thighs and are the most powerful muscle group in the legs. New riders tend to use a stabbing style that produces a jerky transfer to the rear wheel. It's not so much that their downstrokes are wrong, it's that they aren't making a circle by incorporating its other three parts.

2. Bottom. As you reach the bottom of the stroke, concentrate on pulling your foot backward, parallel to the ground. Tour de France winner Greg LeMond described the proper technique perfectly when he said it's like trying to scrape something off the bottom of your shoe. This extends the portion of the pedal stroke in which you can apply power. It's the key to a smooth, fluid transition from the downstroke to the upstroke. It also incorporates the calf and ankle muscles, which distributes the workload and makes the most of your leg strength. You can't come close to pedaling in circles without pulling through at the bottom of the stroke.

Tech Tip

Check any catalog of mountain biking gear, and you'll see an array of shoes. How do you choose? First, narrow it down to the models that work with your clipless pedal system without special inserts or other modifications. The soles must be stiff to block uncomfortable pedal pressure, but not totally rigid, or you won't be able to walk or run well. The tread should look like that of a good hiking boot to provide grip on steep ground. Some shoes come with metal cleats that screw into the soles when you want extra traction. They're helpful when you're scrambling up and down slick slopes, but be careful when walking on rocks and other hard surfaces—you could still slip.

Look for ample protection at the toes for when you bash your feet into hard things. You also want mesh panels or holes along the sides to let out rain or water from stream crossings. It's personal preference whether laces or hook-and-loop straps are better. Some shoes come with both. Hook-and-loop straps are now more durable than in the early days when they got a bad rep for wearing out and failing to hold in wet conditions.

Here's my favorite drill for developing a circular pedal stroke.

While riding on a flat surface, take one foot off its pedal, extend it to the side, and pedal with the other leg. Use a moderately low gear so the resistance won't cause muscle strain. The first time you try this, you won't believe how jerky and inefficient your pedaling is. It feels like you can only make downstrokes because you don't have your other foot pulling up to help you across the top. Ride about 50 yards, then switch feet.

One-legged pedaling will show you exactly how a circular stroke depends on the four components—downstroke, bottom, upstroke, and top. Each must be done correctly and in smooth combination with the others. Practice this drill often enough for the feeling to become ingrained. Try it up a gentle slope, which will make you accentuate the action of driving your knee to the bar. When you return to two-legged pedaling, your stroke will be rounder and more efficient.

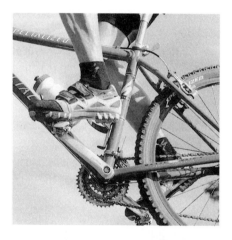 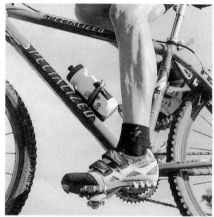

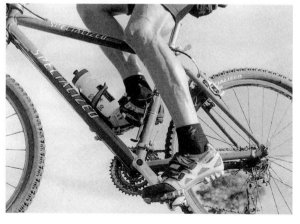

This sequence shows the key elements of a smooth, round, powerful pedal stroke. After you put the muscle to your downstroke (top), *pull your foot through the bottom as if scraping mud from the sole of your shoe* (top right). *By driving your knee toward the handlebar* (bottom), *you help the pedal come up and over the top.*

3. Upstroke. Don't think about pulling up. Except during the slow cadence of a steep climb, your feet move too fast for your brain to keep pace. It's much more effective to simply drive your knee toward the handlebar as soon as your foot passes through the bottom of each

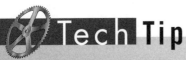

Tech Tip

For performance riding, you need clipless pedals with cleats. This system promotes an efficient pedaling style and improves your control and safety—your foot can't slip off when you're jumping a log, pumping hard up a hill, or rattling on a rough descent. If you're currently riding with loose feet or with toeclips and straps, put a clipless pedal system at the top of your shopping list.

It's tough to recommend a specific brand, because there are at least 10 good ones on the market. Each year, new or improved versions are introduced. All current systems seem to work well and each has its strong supporters. The best advice is to talk with other mountain bikers and with shop mechanics in your area to see what they prefer. Some systems work well in wet climates, for instance, while others tend to more easily become mud-clogged. Some are fine in cold regions, while others, mainly those that use elastomers in their retention hardware, become harder to get into and out of when the temperature drops and the material stiffens.

Whichever pedals you use, for best performance you need to keep them clean and keep their release mechanisms lubricated. Use a "dry" lube that dirt won't stick to. Be careful not to get it on the main surface of the pedals. If there's lube under your cleats, release will be inconsistent—too easy initially, then harder as the lube wears off.

The condition of your cleats also affects release. It's counterintuitive, but as cleats wear down, release actually becomes more difficult. This is because wear isn't consistent across cleats but occurs on certain edges or corners, causing an irregular fit with the pedals. Fresh cleats can make pedals work like new again. Also, check the attachment bolts often. They can vibrate loose, letting the cleats move a bit and messing up the release action.

Forget old-fashioned toeclips and straps for trail riding. They don't keep you tight to the bike and they are actually harder to get into and out of. To remove a foot, you first need to pull back before stepping to the side. With clipless pedals, you simply pivot your heel outward and step down. And because all clipless mountain bike pedals can be engaged from either side, you won't waste time or take your eyes off the trail as you may when trying to turn a toeclip upright.

stroke. Use your powerful hip flexor muscles. If you try to pull up instead of drive forward, the upstroke becomes more vertical, turning your circle into a square. The main objective of the upstroke is to lighten the weight that you're putting on the pedal. This lessens the load for your opposite leg on its downstroke. Studies have shown that it's impossible to pull a pedal up as forcefully as you can push it down. The closer you can come to simply removing weight from the upward pedal, the more efficient and powerful you'll be.

4. Top. The transition from upstroke to downstroke takes care of itself when you've developed the technique of driving your knee toward the handlebar. This pulls your foot through the top with enough momentum to start the downward push. If your opposite foot is doing the right thing—pulling through the bottom—the fluid circle will be complete.

4 Vision

The Eyes Have It

Every technique in this book starts with good vision. I'm not talking only about 20/20 eyesight. In mountain biking, good vision depends on what you're looking at, not just on how well you see it. The reason is integral to bike control. Just as a ball bearing rolls to a magnet, your wheels will tend to go right to the spot on which your eyes are focused.

As you read through this book, you'll find several stories about what happens when you look at a place where you *don't* want to go. You need to focus your vision on the gaps between rocks, not on the rocks themselves. Look at the edge of the trail, not at what's over the edge—or you'll probably get a much closer view than you want.

The second rule of good vision is to scan farther ahead the faster you go. If you're always looking right in front of your wheel, you won't be able to plan the fastest, safest, and most efficient line. You won't have time to adjust your body position, steering inputs, and pedaling. The result will be frustrating mistakes that make it very hard to ever reach your trail-riding potential.

But wait a minute—don't you need to look down at that gap between rocks when you get to it? Not really. It's not going anywhere. You'll find that once you've established the correct line, you can keep scanning past the immediate section and your wheels will stay on track. A quick glance down is

21

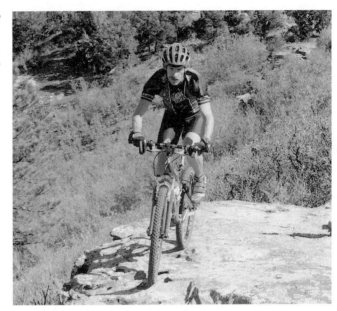

Keep your eyes trained on the line you want, not on things that you want to avoid (like the cliff on my right). A bike has an uncanny way of going right to the place at which you look.

okay as long as it's *quick*. Until you get the hang of it, it may be hard to re-sist sneaking a peek, but the faster you're going, the more you need to look ahead. The ideal technique is to use just your peripheral vision for close ob-jects so you can watch for things farther up the trail.

Good vision also means seeing ruts in time to be off the brakes when you reach them. It means seeing smooth spots so you can grab the brakes and scrub off speed before you reach a turn or rocky section. It means spot-ting a bump or dip in time to suck it up so you won't be launched into the air and unable to make your next move. It means recognizing an off-camber turn in time to put out your inside foot to use as an outrigger. Good vision is your key to fluid riding, relaxation, and confidence.

Whipping the Enemies
of Good Vision

I've competed many times with a ton of mud in my eyes, but one race stands out. It's kind of a funny story, although I didn't think so back then. It was actually one of the first big events I ever rode, an autumn race in New England sponsored by the old Ross bike company. A cold rain set in just be-fore the start. For the first 90 minutes, I barely noticed the miserable conditions as the intensity of my effort kept me warm. But then I ran out of energy. The combination of hard riding, bonking, and bone-chilling cold really hammered me in the last half-hour.

What put me over the edge, though, was the sandy, wet soil that was being thrown up by my front tire. I had long ago jettisoned my glasses because it was impossible to see through them. Now the sand was slopping into my eyeballs. My eyelids were wiping it down and packing it in. By the end of the race, my vision was totally blurred. Every blink felt like sandpaper. I couldn't see, my energy was gone, and I was so cold I could no longer control the bike.

My older sister had come to watch her first bike race. When she found me later at the motel, I was in the bathtub. What a sight—I was still wearing all of my riding clothes, including my shoes. As I lay there, shivering uncontrollably in the muddy water, I wondered if I had permanently damaged my vision. My sister took one look and suggested that I might just be a moron to be pursuing a pro cycling career.

Even though I rinsed my eyes as best I could, there was still lots of stuff packed into them. For the next couple of mornings, I woke up with mud oozing from the corners of my eyes.

Although that race was an extreme situation, it's certainly not the only time my vision has been hampered. In muddy conditions, just seeing the trail well enough to ride the right line is half the challenge.

In a race, you can't afford the time it takes to stop and wipe stuff out of your eyes. Often, you can't even risk taking a hand off the bar. You need to blink the junk to the bottom or side as you keep riding. On training or recreational rides, you can and should stop. Continuing while your vision is impaired can result in a needless crash.

Things happen fast on a technical trail. You need clear, sharp, unobstructed vision to ride your best. You'll find specific vision tips with each technique throughout the book. Here is some other guidance to help you maintain good vision.

Sunglasses. In muddy races like the one I just described, you can start with sunglasses but they'll soon become too mucked up to see through. Instead of taking them off, try to retain some protection by sliding them to the end of your nose. Then you can look over the top of the glasses and they can still block some of the mud that comes up from the front wheel. If it's bumpy, though, they aren't likely to stay on long when they're perched out there.

Unless you're using cheap disposable sunglasses (not a bad idea for racing, as long as they're shatterproof), try to remember the spot where you take them off if you're forced to jettison them. If you're lucky, you can find them afterward. At one rainy event at California's Big Bear, it looked like a factory closeout sale at the top of a descent. It was so slippery that guys didn't even want to risk reaching around to put their grimy glasses into their pockets. In a race where you know your sunglasses are going to get plastered or lost, a friend can give you a clean pair when you reach the designated hand-up area on each lap.

The problem is not only what your front tire is sending up but also what other riders are flinging at you from all directions. Knobby tires pick up rocks as well as dirt and mud. It's hard to imagine any good reason for not wearing eye protection, though some people do ride without it. Personally, I think that's foolish.

You'll find sports sunglasses with lenses tinted to almost any color. Some models come with several lenses that you can quickly interchange. Clear, light amber, or rose works well in most conditions, as opposed to darker hues that can be a problem in shady sections. Dark lenses increase the time that your eyes need to adjust when moving from sunlight to shade. Make sure the lenses you use for cycling are shatterproof and block ultraviolet light.

Helmet visor. Almost every helmet that's marketed for off-road riding comes with a detachable visor, or you can buy one to add on. In sunny conditions, a visor keeps the glare out of your eyes and shades your face from sunburn. On a wet trail, it can block some of the stuff that's flung at you by the wheels of other riders. Your glasses will stay cleaner.

There's a downside to using a visor, though. Because it cuts off your upward vision, you're in greater danger of being whacked in the head by low-hanging branches. Some serious accidents have happened this way. You can get clotheslined right off your bike. Beware of this danger. It may be safer to remove your visor on rides in the woods or at least to use the type that pops off when it catches onto something.

Sweat catcher. Glasses can get just as messed up on the inside as on the outside. That's why one company's attempt to make mountain biking glasses with tear-off lenses didn't work. Sure, you could peel away the side covered by external slop, but you still couldn't see through the streaks and condensation on the inside.

The main cause of this problem is the sweat or rain that runs down from your forehead. In dry conditions, sweat combines with dust to create a coating that's very tough to see through. One way to stop the waterfall is to wear a sweatband under your helmet. For me, this works only for awhile on a hot or humid day. Eventually, the sweatband gets so soaked that it starts drooling down my glasses. I've tried using thicker bands that hold more moisture, but when you hit a big bump, they can let loose like a dam breaking. Still, in most conditions, a sweatband is the most effective way I know to keep glasses streak-free.

Corrective lenses. I don't need corrective lenses for cycling, but I know a number of riders who do. Most prefer contact lenses to glasses, because there's less risk of problems. If you ride with contacts, carry a little bottle of saline solution for an emergency eye flush if something gets under a lens. If you can't wear contacts, most makers of sports sunglasses can grind your prescription into one of their models. There's always the risk, though, that glasses will get bounced off, broken in a crash, or fouled by sweat, mud, rain, or spray.

Crud catcher. This is a lightweight piece of plastic that you can attach to your bike just before a wet ride or race. It mounts under the frame's down tube with zip-ties or hook-and-loop straps for easy installation and removal. It's long enough and wide enough to block a lot of the mud and water flung up by the front wheel. I always install one for a muddy race.

5 Shifting

Change Your Gears Early and Often

Mountain bike technology has come a long way in a short while, but it hasn't come quite far enough. Despite all the advancements in frames, suspensions, and wheels, we're still saddled with an archaic way of changing gears. Sure, today's shifters are quicker and more accurate, but they still work by pushing the chain back and forth to different sprockets just as bikes have for the last half-century.

This is the bicycle's weak link. The derailleurs, with their exposed pivots and pulleys, get blasted by the elements and damaged by rocks, branches, and crashes. Meanwhile, the cables and chain get gunked up with mud or dirt, and their lubrication gets washed away in water crossings. Even when the drivetrain is perfectly clean, there's still lots of friction as the long chain wraps around the sprockets and winds through the pulleys.

Well, there's no use complaining. Nothing better is on the horizon. The right approach is to help these antique parts work as well as possible by keeping them clean, lubricated, and adjusted. After that, it's all a matter of honing your shifting technique.

Proper Planning

Your mountain bike has 21, 24, or 27 gears (3 chainrings multiplied by 7, 8, or 9 cogs). Almost every gear is usable except perhaps the smallest cog in combination with the little chainring. The chain has minimal tension in this position and its angle may cause the links to rattle against the middle ring. In general, though, you should be able to find the right gear for nearly every section of every trail. "Right" simply means a ratio that lets you keep the crankarms turning no matter what resistance you encounter.

To ride with the magic combination of speed and finesse, you need to anticipate shifts. You want to make them when your cadence, or pedal rpm, is relatively high and your pedaling force is low. This makes efficient use of your energy and helps your derailleurs operate as reliably as they can.

The goal, always, is to maintain momentum. This is especially important in rolling or hilly terrain, where shifts are frequent and often take place on climbs. You want to upshift to higher gears in time to prevent your legs from spinning ineffectively against light resistance. Upshifts aren't difficult to time and goofs aren't costly, so most riders don't have a problem. Conversely, if you downshift too soon, your legs will flail with too high a cadence and your speed will drop. If you downshift too late, you'll lose both leg speed and forward speed, and waste energy as you push against too much resistance.

Downshifting Dilemmas

Downshifts are where the greatest chance of mistakes occurs, particularly with the front derailleur. When shifting to a smaller chainring, almost all derailleurs pull the chain down with spring action. You release cable tension with the shift lever, which lets a spring move the derailleur cage inward over a smaller ring. The hang up (literally) comes when you fail to downshift until you're too far into a hill. By then, you're pedaling hard to keep momentum, which stretches the chain tight around the chainring. So tight, in fact, that the cage can't pull it off and drop it down. At this point, you must relax your pedaling force until the chain derails. On any decent grade, this will instantly scrub off speed. If the guy next to you anticipates his shift and makes it before being forced to lighten pedal pressure, well, enjoy the chase.

As you may already have discovered, when you try to downshift with a heavy pedal load, you can encounter another big problem: chainsuck. This nasty-sounding thing happens when the chain does shift from the middle to small chainring but is under too much pressure to release from the middle ring's teeth. It gets pulled up and wedged against the chainstay, freezing the crankset instantly. Not only is this harmful to all the equipment involved but it also stops you dead. This is why you'll find my main discussion of chainsuck in chapter 11, Momentum. You prevent chainsuck the

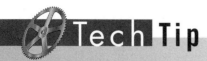

Tech Tip

Here's how to adjust a conventional rear derailleur so it will shift trouble-free. (*Note:* In the fall of 1998, Shimano introduced models that move opposite of the way this describes. The adjustment principles are the same, but cable tension is reversed for upshifts and downshifts.)

Find the two limit screws in the derailleur body. Usually they're marked "L" and "H" for low and high gear. They adjust the derailleur's travel to the biggest and smallest cogs, respectively.

With your bike in a workstand, try shifts across the range of cogs. I recommend setting the limit screws as tight as possible while still allowing the chain to complete shifts to the biggest and smallest cogs. Any extra travel may produce good shifting on the workstand, but under heavy pedaling loads on rough trails, you may get a damaging overshift.

Shifts to in-between cogs should be crisp in each direction. If the chain balks at climbing to bigger cogs, turn the cable adjustment barrel (where the cable enters the derailleur) one-half turn counterclockwise until the problem is corrected. If shifts to smaller cogs are balky, turn the barrel clockwise.

A front derailleur can be installed or adjusted with the bike in a workstand, but the job isn't complete until you test it while riding. Things may not work the same way when the chain has a pedaling load.

To test the setting of the high-gear (H) limit screw, put the chain on a small cog in back, then shift from the small to big chainring under different pedaling loads. Really throw the chain up there. If it falls to the outside of the big ring, tighten the limit screw one-quarter turn and re-test. It the big ring won't quite pick up the chain, back off the limit screw by one-quarter turns until it does.

Check the shift to the small ring (adjusted by the L screw). This shift requires the spring in the derailleur to overcome tension on the chain. If you're in the middle of a steep hill, pedaling with great force, the derailleur won't shift, regardless of how far the limit screw is backed off. That's why you must ease off pedal pressure for a revolution while downshifting on a climb. Correct derailleur adjustment will let the chain be pulled to the small ring but not past it and down around the bottom bracket. Make sure the derailleur cage moves inward just enough to prevent the chain from rattling against it in the granny gear (the small-chainring/big-cog combination).

Chain length is the final mechanical requirement for good shifting. For best performance, I recommend the shortest chain that still lets you shift in and out of the big-ring/big-cog crossover gear.

29

same way you avoid rejected downshifts—by shifting only under light-to-moderate pedal pressure.

There's a way to downshift the rear derailleur efficiently, too. I recall dueling with fellow pro racer Tinker Juarez at a World Cup race in Park City, Utah. He was strong that day and climbing great, so he was gapping me at the top of every hill. We reached a series of rollers, which was going to spell the end for me if I didn't concentrate on my shifting. I pedaled down each hill and through the bottom to build momentum, then I started downshifting with a high cadence to get up the next grade. Click, click, click—one gear at a time at just the right moment, up over the top and down to the next bottom, where I caught Tinker again. This happened on four or five consecutive hills.

By shifting smoothly and pedaling evenly, I made the most of my energy, while Tinker was not so conscientious. The climbs proved he was stronger, but I counteracted his strength with my gears. I didn't let him build a lead. By the end, he wore down, allowing me to get away and win the race.

Perpetual Pedaling

In order to shift gears, you must be pedaling. Seems obvious, right? Don't assume that most riders understand this, though. At least, they don't practice it. What I'm referring to here is developing the habit of pedaling almost continuously instead of coasting frequently, especially while descending.

Again, it's a matter of preserving precious momentum. Keep your legs turning and change gears as often as necessary to maintain a moderate pedal resistance. If you usually coast down hills and resume pedaling somewhere along the way, the chances are real good that you won't be in the right gear. In fact, you may almost be out of control if the bike is bouncing and your legs are flailing because the gear is too small. Instead, shift up to a bigger gear as the downhill begins and continue pedaling (at least intermittently) as you descend. This will help you be in the right gear at the bottom so you can carry momentum into the flats or up the next hill.

Always maintain pedaling when approaching a climb. If you coast in, you increase the chance that when you resume pedaling you'll be in a gear that's too large. Then you bog down. Your bike has as many as 27 gears, so use them all and change them often. When you do it right, it's like having an automatic transmission. Just as you sense too much resistance, downshift to the next-largest cog to regain the right pedal pressure. Do it again and again until you're over the top, then upshift to higher gears in the same way. When you're turning the crankset, you're riding the bike. When you're coasting, you're just along for the ride.

Multi-Cog Shifts

Ideally, your fine sense of anticipation won't put you into situations where you need to shift across several cogs at a time. But occasionally, this is unavoidable, for instance, when you round a tight bend and are greeted by a wall.

Whenever a multi-cog gear change is necessary, ease your pedal pressure at the instant of the shift to prevent an incapacitating derailleur jam. This is the same pedaling technique used to assist front downshifts on climbs. It's often easier said than done, though, especially in race situations where you may not be thinking clearly. You come into a hill and, instead of progressively working through the cogs, you suddenly need to grab a handful. The rear end of the bike just detonates—the derailleur is over here, the chain is over there, and you're not going anywhere until you stop to sort it out.

Shimano's Rapid Rise shifters prevent this because they make you downshift one cog at a time. You can't pulverize things when going into a hill. It takes about half of a pedal revolution for each gear change, so it's slower than a single shift across three or four cogs, but it eliminates the risk. Personally, I'm not a big fan of this system. When racing, I want the option of jumping over several cogs to handle an abrupt change in the trail. To me, the advantage is worth the risk.

Sometimes, you bog down and need to shift both derailleurs. Which one first? Always the front. The rear can downshift under a heavy load but the front never will. Shift from the big ring to the middle or from the middle to the small, then start working your way to larger cogs.

Break This Rule

Everything you read and everyone you listen to will warn against using the big-chainring/big-cog combination. This is called a crossover gear because it angles the chain quite severely from front to back and stretches it tightly around the two largest sprockets. Conventional wisdom says that this results in extra friction and wear to the chain and teeth.

There's no question about these consequences. Even so, the big/big combo is my favorite gear, and I recommend that you use it, too—but only when the time is right and you don't stay in it too long.

31

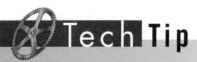

So when is it cool to crossover? Let's say you're in the big ring, jamming hard, and you come to a short hill. You need a lower gear, but the last thing you want is to lose momentum by backing off pedal pressure to make a shift to the middle ring. Besides, in many cases the ratio reduction from switching chainrings will be more than you need, slowing you even more. Instead, stay in the big ring, keep powering the pedals, and shift to larger cogs—even to the largest one. Rear shifts are way faster than front shifts, and mis-shifts aren't nearly as likely.

There is one catch, though. You must make sure your chain is long enough to get in and out of the big/big combo. Remember, it wraps the maximum amount of chain around sprockets. Even if you choose not to use this gear intentionally, you may shift into it absentmindedly. You may get in, but you won't get out.

I saw a classic example of this in the Sea Otter Classic cross-country race. Cadel Evans of the Australian Olympic team, was at the front of a five-man group, forcing the pace. I was at my limit, barely able to hang on. Suddenly, Cadel was off his bike, trying to figure out a problem. As I rode by, I saw his rear derailleur stretched to the limit, his chain locked into the big/big combo. I smiled because it moved me up one place—a place I had earned, having learned that lesson 10 years before. These days, I don't get stuck in the crossover gear, I just use it to my advantage.

6 Tire Traction

Where the Tread Meets the Trail

In our look at momentum in chapter 11, I'll give you lots of advice to keep your tires gripping on various surfaces—mud, sand, gravel, snow, ice, and even water. In fact, good traction is so essential to off-road riding that you'll find tips popping up throughout this book. When you get right down to it, a key measure of any rider's skill is his ability to find traction and then hang on to it.

But there's more to it than skill. Tire selection can make or break your ability to ride certain surfaces well (or even at all). Put an excellent rider on treads that are unsuited to a particular trail, and he'll be frustrated with his performance. Conversely, put an average rider on the ideal rubber for the conditions, and he'll be able to milk the most from his ability. That's how important the right tires are.

"Okay," I hear you saying, "so tell me which tires to use." I said the same thing to many tire experts. Unfortunately, I got back about as many different answers as people I talked to. There are numerous tread-design theories in the tire industry as well as a wide selection of rubber compounds for wet or dry conditions. Combine these with the array of soils and riding styles, and selecting the best tire becomes sort of like selecting the best wine. What works for me may not please you at all, and the next guy will prefer something else entirely.

There are so many performance characteristics to consider—climbing traction, braking traction, cornering traction, and rolling resistance, to name the four major ones. Obviously, one tire can't be the best at everything. There must be trade-offs. The result is dozens of tread designs, some of which strive to give decent all-around performance, while others try for an edge in specific conditions.

Tread Trade-Offs

One trend has been toward bald tires with minimal tread. Because the knobs are short and so widely spaced, you lose some climbing, braking, and cornering traction, but you benefit from lower rolling resistance. You get a bigger, smoother contact patch (the section in touch with the ground).

On most dry trails, this works pretty well, but these tires require more finesse to ride. If you brake too hard, they lock up and skid. If you don't have your weight over the rear wheel when climbing, they lose traction more quickly.

What you get for these negative attributes is more speed. These tires are fast. I like them best on damp or loamy dirt—surfaces that by their nature provide lots of traction to make up for the tires' weak grip. In the wet, though, it's a different story. Bald treads lose traction much too quickly on mud.

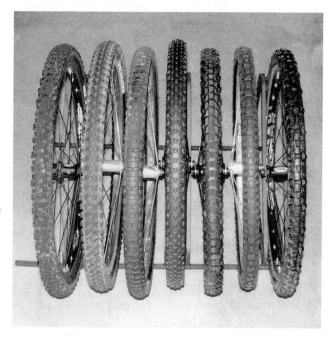

Tires come with an amazing variety of tread designs, so the trick is to determine which works best in your terrain. Narrow it down by checking which tread is on the wheels of experienced local riders. The third tire from the right is an example of a "bald" tread with the smoother, faster center that is preferred by some racers.

Speaking of short knobs, that is another trend of tread evolution. Some tires still have knobs all over them like in the old days, but now the knobs are shorter so they flex less and rolling resistance is minimized. Less rubber also means less weight, always an advantage in wheels. The trade-off is that the treads will wear down sooner, and even when they're new, they won't provide as much traction as taller knobs in certain mud or soft-dirt conditions.

Knobby Knowledge

Personally, give me knobs, but not big knobs. I'm amazed that the Europeans so often race on nearly bald treads. To me, the traction is inadequate on most surfaces. Short knobs give me better grip and better steering control because they're predictable.

I also gravitate toward tires with rounder profiles. I find that they steer easier and corner quicker than those that are flatter across the top. A flat profile can be unpredictable, especially if the side knobs are not well-supported. Once you get on the tires' edges during a corner, the knobs tend to roll over. Square edges also make it harder to pull moves like riding up and out of a steep-sided rut that's parallel to the trail. Tires with rounder, more gradual transitions from top to sides work well in the usual variety of conditions. They also have a lower rolling resistance than tires with flatter profiles.

Other important factors include tire width, knob configurations, and rubber compounds (softer for better grip or harder for greater durability). Wider tires give you bigger contact patches for better traction. However, wider also means more rolling resistance and potential clearance problems with the frame. In muddy conditions, there can be major buildup around the brakes, under the fork, and between the chainstays behind the bottom bracket. If the tires fill most of the space, these areas can quickly become so jammed with mud that the wheels will hardly turn. Generally, good mud tires have knobs that aren't too tall or closely spaced, so mud is flung away rather than collected. Such tread patterns often are referred to as self-cleaning.

Tire widths range from about 1.5 to 2.5 inches. Besides the pros and cons that I've mentioned, wider tires have one other characteristic: more shock absorption. You can safely run lower inflation pressure so the tires will cushion impacts and increase comfort. This is a nice benefit for recreational mountain biking, though racers don't want the trade-off—greater rolling resistance and slightly slower steering response.

Compared to narrow tires, wide ones let you decrease air pressure by a

Ned's KNOWLEDGE

Once you've determined the best tire to race on, train on it, too. That's the only way to learn its handling characteristics. But there's a catch: You also need to use the same inflation pressure during training that you do when racing.

I see so many guys who let their tires go soft during the week. They might even bleed air to make training rides more comfortable. Then race day comes. They pump up to the psi that gives them fast bikes with low rolling resistance, but they don't feel confident on them. The bikes behave differently. Traction decreases. Their wheels break loose sooner in corners and chatter to the outside in bumpy turns.

The result is easy to imagine. These riders can't perform as well as they should. When you blast down a hill on 48 psi instead of on 35 psi, you'll know what I mean. Your control decreases as your tire pressure (and speed) increases.

The only way to become good on hard, fast tires is to train on them. Make sure inflation stays constant by checking your tires with a pressure gauge before each ride. Your training rides won't be as comfortable (unless you're on a dual-suspension bike), but you'll reap the rewards on race day.

few psi without a huge increase in the risk of an internal puncture called a pinch flat. A pinch flat happens when a sharp impact causes the tube to be squeezed between the tire and rim, resulting in two little holes that sometimes are called a snakebite. A wider tire has more bulk to prevent the tube from being pinched. The lower the pressure in any tire, though, the greater the risk of a pinch flat.

I usually race on 1.9-inch tires. I like 45 psi in front and 48 in back. At my weight, 145 pounds, that's pretty high air pressure. It's my insurance against getting pinch flats when going fast. If you're heavier, you may need even more pressure. There's no formula for how much. Your weight, suspension setup, trail conditions, and ability to unweight over obstacles will determine the psi you need. Experience is the best guide. When you reach the point where pinch flats are virtually eliminated but bike control isn't impaired, you have it. Then each time you ride, use a pressure gauge (rather than merely squeezing the tire with your hand) to make sure the inflation is exactly right.

For recreational trail riding, 35 to 40 psi should be plenty. You'll find that most tires have good traction and are predictable in this range. Dual suspension lets you run a few pounds less if you want an even plusher ride. I don't recommend inflation under 30 psi, however. You'll feel a dropoff in rolling efficiency and handling, and you'll risk more snakebites than Indiana Jones in a den of cobras.

Puncture Pointers

Punctures are certainly the most common mechanical problem in mountain biking. In most cases, fixing a flat means replacing the tube rather than actually patching it (at least until you get back home). It can be a hassle to find and patch a hole beside the trail, especially in wet conditions. Instead, pack at least one extra tube, and carry a patch kit for those times when punctures outnumber your spares.

I rarely get a flat tire—probably because I'm light and so finicky about running enough tire pressure—but most racers get lots of them. At a race, they preride the course and their inflation seems fine, but they aren't going at race speed. When the competitive juices are flowing and they blast into rocky sections, they pinch flat all over the place. The most proficient flat-fixers (because they get to practice a lot) can replace a front tube in a couple of minutes and take maybe three minutes to fix the rear. I've seen my friend Steve Tilford, who has been racing (and flatting) since pre-suspension days, replace a front tube and get riding again inside of 90 seconds.

That's fast, but it's still a lot of time to give to your competition, so I believe that avoiding flats is priority one. Then, when bad luck happens, it pays to have your supplies organized and your flat-fixing technique sharply honed. If you're a racer, I strongly recommend practicing at home. Use a stopwatch. The time you save could win you a race someday. Here's the procedure for a rear flat (not all steps are required for a front, of course).

1. Shift the rear derailleur to the smallest cog before you stop. If you can't, hand pedal to this gear when you jump off. This moves the derailleur out from under the cassette for easier wheel removal. You'll also know where to place the chain so everything lines up properly when you reinstall the wheel. Make it easier to get going again by having the chain on the middle chainring, or even on the granny ring if you're on a climb. (If you have a Grip Shift rear derailleur, put the chain on the largest cog for wheel removal, rather than on the smallest. Spring tension makes it hard to reinstall the wheel when the chain is on the smallest cog.)

2. Remove the supplies from your seatbag or jersey pocket.

3. Release the brake so the pads open wide for tire clearance.

4. Open the hub's quick-release.

5. Remove the wheel by pulling the derailleur back with your right hand as you push the wheel forward and down with your left. Lay the bike on its left side so the drivetrain is off the ground.

6. Depress the valve to release any remaining air.

7. Pull one edge (the bead) of the tire off the rim all the away around. Use a tire lever, if necessary. You'll save time if you avoid tires that fit so tightly on your brand of rims that you need to use a tire lever to re-move them.

8. Reach in on the opposite side of the wheel from the valve stem, grab the tube, and pull it out.

9. Quickly feel around the inner circumference of the tire, even if you're positive that the tube has a pinch flat. You need to be certain that there isn't something sharp stuck through the tread. If there is and you don't get it out, the new tube will immediately be punctured. Also check for a rip in the tire sidewall. Flats from this type of damage are usually sudden blowouts rather than slow leaks. You need to patch or cover the rip, or the new tube will blow out, too.

10. Add just enough air to the new tube to unflatten it. With a presta valve, the quickest way is to unscrew it then blow with your mouth. This won't work with a Schrader valve, so you'll need to use your pump or CO_2 cartridge.

11. Put the valve through the rim hole, then feed the tube into the tire all the way around. Push the tire bead back onto the rim with your thumbs or the heels of your hands. If you need a tire lever to pry the last section onto the rim, get tires that don't fit your rims so tightly. Using a lever can pinch a hole in the new tube, especially when you're rushing the job to get back in the race.

12. Inflate the tire to the point where thumb pressure tells you it's right. Use a CO_2 cartridge during a race. The fill is instant and doesn't waste en-ergy like using a hand pump. Go easy on the gas until you're sure the tire is correctly seated. Check that the tube isn't bulging between the bead and the rim.

13. Reinstall the wheel. Make sure it's centered, then close the hub quick-release and the brake. (On bikes with tight clearance between the brake pads, you may need to reinstall the wheel before you inflate the tire. Figure this out during practice, not on the race course.)

14. Don't leave the scene before jamming the bad tube, CO_2 cartridge, and other paraphernalia into your seatbag or jersey pocket. It's okay to leave stuff on a race course if you're certain it will be cleaned up later, but on recreational rides remember the International Mountain Bicycling Association rule and "leave no trace."

Race-Day Strategies

In competition, I often carry two spare tubes and two CO_2 cartridges. I pack one tube and cartridge in my seatbag and the others in my jersey pocket. My seatbag also contains a tire lever, just in case. (Also in there are a chain tool, and a multitool with screwdriver blades and 4-, 5-, and 6-mm allen keys. On training rides, I pack a patch kit, too.)

Be sure to secure all of these items. I frequently see guys open their seatbags and find nothing but garbage. Loose tools can quickly wear a hole through a tube, and the tools themselves can be damaged from rattling together. And who wants to hear all that noise? Another scenario is discovering that the bag somehow opened and jettisoned its contents along the trail. Prevent this by putting the zipper's tab under a strap so it can't work open. Then use an old toe strap to make the bag doubly secure under the saddle.

During a race, you're usually up against tough conditions when you stop for a flat. Your heart is pounding, sweat is running into your eyes, and your hands are wet and muddy. It helps a lot if you've packed the spare tube without its box and removed the little round knurled nut at the base of the valve stem (on presta tubes only). It can be hard to unscrew this nut with slippery fingers. I've even heard of cases where nuts were cross-threaded at the factory and wouldn't budge. Imagine whipping out your spare tube and discovering that. Unscrew the metal presta valve cap so the tube is ready for air, then screw the plastic valve cap over the valve for protection. Carefully fold the tube and wrap it in an old sock or plastic bag if it's the one that's going into the seatbag. Just put a rubber band around it if it'll be carried in your pocket.

Sometimes, a tire develops a slow leak rather than loses all of its air at once. When this happens in a race, keep riding. It wastes time to stop and sit by the trail with your finger on the valve before you can begin the tube replacement. Instead, stay on the bike until most of the air is out. Another advantage is that riding on a soft tire loosens it on the rim, making it easier to get the bead off. On rocky ground, don't wait too long to stop, because the risk of rim damage goes up as the tire goes down.

If you're concerned about performance, don't try to reduce punctures by switching to thick tubes. They're heavy, and I don't think they're any

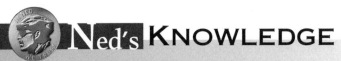

Ned's KNOWLEDGE

It was a national points series race in Indiana. Torrential rain before the start left the course oozing with slimy mud. Traction was only a dream. Guys were spinning out everywhere.

On the main climb, I was riding one gear higher than normal and trying my best to pedal in smooth circles. My weight was way back on the saddle and my torso was upright to help the rear tire grab whatever it could. This lightened the front wheel so much that the bike seemed to be taking me where it wanted to go instead of where I wanted to go.

Then on the downhill, I discovered a small muddy berm created by all the passing wheels. By staying just to the inside, I rode much more confidently, even though my handlebar was almost debarking the trees. I was passing guys and using less energy at the same time.

That was about the time when the rear tire punctured. It was a slow leak, so I continued riding. The softening tire actually helped traction for awhile.

What a mess when I stopped. Mud was covering the wheel and my seatbag. I was sweating like crazy. The woods were dark. And to top it off, I had an audience. A group of spectators just happened to be right there.

One guy started driving me nuts with his small talk, asking me how I was feeling, how I liked Indiana, you name it. I had to catch myself to keep from telling him to shut up. Instead, I said (not very politely), "Let me focus on fixing this." After I finally got the tube in and the tire on, I reached for my CO_2 cartridge. It had disappeared, camouflaged by the mud and leaves. I was going crazy when the same guy whom I almost told to shut up said, "There it is."

I had to smile. I had been so ticked off at this guy, and now he had saved me. I said, "Thanks, pal," aired up my tire, rejoined the race, and made it back to fifth place by the finish.

The moral of this story: Be nice to spectators (or keep your stuff in your pocket till you need it).

more flat-resistant. In fact, I recommend getting the weight-saving advantages of ultralight tubes. Anything that flats one of them will probably puncture a heavier tube as well.

In areas where thorns are a big problem, race with tubes that contain sealant. The goo is pretty heavy but it does a good job of plugging thorn-size punctures before any significant amount of air is lost. You can buy tubes with sealant already inside, called airlock tubes, or you can put your own sealant into standard tubes. I prefer adding my own so I can save weight by using the minimum amount. Sealant is sold in bike shops or auto-parts stores.

Tire liners are another solution in thorny areas. These strips lie inside the circumference of the tire to stop sharp things from penetrating as far as the tube. Again, you want to minimize weight, so go for the thin liners made of Kevlar rather than for the thicker plastic ones.

Flats sometimes result from tire sidewall damage rather than from an actual puncture. Once a sidewall is cut or torn, it lets the tube protrude and blow out. Your spare tube will suffer the same fate unless you line the inside of the damaged area. In a pinch, you can use an energy bar wrapper or a dollar bill (which is pretty strong because it's actually linen, not paper). I prefer duct tape because it's tough and sticks in place. I keep some wrapped around the tire lever in my seatbag. You can make it through a race or ride with a repaired sidewall, but beware when descending, because it could blow out again. Replace the tire before your next ride.

Rim strips are the final consideration. They protect the tubes from internal punctures caused by the ends of the spokes or sharp edges left by the rim manufacturer. Some wheels come with plastic rim strips, and sometimes shops or mechanics use strapping tape. Take it from a guy who lost a national championship three miles from the finish because of a rim strip–related flat tire: Be safe and use Velox rim tape. All the other materials can loosen, move, or wear through. French-made Velox is a thick, strong cotton with an adhesive backing to keep it in place. It removes one very frustrating puncture producer from the list.

No matter what you do to prevent flats, you'll still get one now and then. When it happens in a race, don't be discouraged and quit. Have what you need to make the repair, be well-practiced, and keep your head. If you make a quick repair, you can get back in without losing many places. And who knows—guys in front may flat, and you'll be right back in the prizes. It takes a lot of time, energy, and money to travel to races. Don't let flats knock you out.

7 Braking

Use Your Stoppers for More Safety, Control—and Speed

Mountain biking is so physically demanding that riders tend to train for leg strength and cardiovascular ability while ignoring less obvious necessities. But consider what you go through two hours into a ride or race. It's not just your engine that suffers—it's your driving ability, too. Braking is one of the most important skills to keep intact.

How important? Consider what happened at the Hunter Mountain World Cup race in upstate New York. It was raining. The main descent was a radically steep minefield of rocks covered with a thin layer of mud. On the first lap, I made it down in good shape. But as I became more fatigued, I couldn't relax my forearms. I couldn't squeeze the brakes hard enough to slow down quickly in the opportune places, so I had to apply them all the time. This made my arms even more tired. I was on the edge of losing control. After narrowly missing some trees, I surrendered and began running down the hill each lap.

On and Off

The right way to get down the hill, if I could have managed it, would have been to squeeze the brakes hard for short bursts and then release them.

Here's another way to think of it. Coaches talk about a no-man's-land in training—that middle intensity that's too hard to allow recovery but not hard enough to make you faster. Braking should be viewed like that. Either brake hard or get off the brakes completely. On long downhills, if you constantly contract your forearm muscles by pulling the levers, there's no chance to relax. Your arms will fatigue and you'll lose strength and maneuverability. But when you brake in an on/off fashion, your forearm muscles get periods to rest and recover.

Lots of riders think that they get off the brakes, but they still drag them lightly. They're on them hard, then stay on them soft. Here's my check: When I go down a hill, I want to hear my levers click open against the stops. This ensures that the pads are completely off the rims. Another trick is to periodically extend each hand's two braking fingers (index and middle) straight ahead, off the levers.

The key to fast downhills is to put the brakes on hard in areas where there's adequate braking traction, then let go of the levers when riding over loose rocks, roots, ruts, or other irregular surfaces. Just 3 smooth feet can give you enough traction to scrub off a lot of speed. If you're racing on a lap course, you can remember the smooth spots and use them each time around.

Ideally, you'll be able to do most braking with the front wheel. It has the most stopping power, especially when you can get your weight back and drive that tire into the ground. But be careful. When using the front brake hard, you need to keep your body vertical. Don't brake hard in a turn, or the result could very well be a front-wheel washout and heavy crash. Get on the brake when you're in proper alignment on a smooth patch, then get off as you turn or chatter through rough or loose sections.

The rear brake is less effective than the front, but it's still useful. It can help you scrub off speed in situations like the one I've just described, where it's risky to use the front brake. It's easy to unintentionally lock the rear wheel as your weight transfers forward, but this type of skid rarely results in a wholesale loss of control and a crash. By keeping your body low and your weight back, you'll improve rear-wheel traction and reduce skidding.

Downhill Technique

You need to brake on most steep downhills to control your speed, but this also is the riskiest time to touch those levers. Sometimes, braking in an attempt to prevent a crash can actually cause one. A classic example is when you panic a bit and hit your front brake hard without first putting your weight back. With such a high center of gravity, you pitch forward—maybe right over the handlebar. To prevent this, always descend steep grades with your body pushed way back. Don't lock your elbows straight, though. You still need some bend to absorb shock and maintain steering control.

To get any bite at all with the rear brake, you need to have your butt over the rear wheel. In fact, on a really steep descent, your saddle should be under your stomach. Practice getting into and out of this position. If you're a newcomer, it will help to lower the saddle several inches so you can move back and forth more freely. This boosts confidence because it's easier to get back onto the saddle. You can't stop to adjust saddle height in a race, of course, but it makes practicing less intimidating until you get the hang of it.

When you get a chance to watch a downhill race, you'll see competitors with their seats as much as four inches lower than they'd have them for cross-country riding. This allows them to have a very low, very rearward position for braking control at critical points on the course. They then stand and sprint on the pedaling sections. Cross-country racers can't be as specialized with positions, but the general technique is the same.

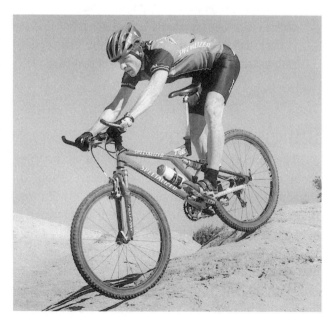

To prevent tipping forward into an endo when braking on steep descents, keep your upper body low and way back. This puts your weight behind the front wheel and over the rear wheel, increasing braking traction at both ends.

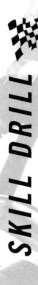

It's a fact that the front brake is stronger than the rear. For this reason, lots of riders are reluctant to use it, probably because they fear an endo—going over the front wheel. Here's a drill to get you comfortable with your front brake's stopping power. The key is making a rearward weight shift.

Find a short, smooth downhill with a clear runout at the bottom. Place a rock to designate the braking point on the runout. Start at the same place on the hill for each run. Coast, don't pedal, so you'll reach the identical speed each time and be able to compare stopping distances. First, apply only the front brake as you pass the rock. Make sure to stay vertical with the bike (don't turn the handlebar), or the front tire will lose traction and slide out. Extend your arms to push your weight back. Be careful the first time so you don't endo. Modulate the lever to prevent locking the wheel and skidding. Mark the spot where you stop. Repeat several times to achieve the shortest distance possible.

Next, use only the rear brake for several runs and mark your stopping points. Finally, use both brakes. Compare distances. The first thing you should realize is how much power you have in the front brake. The difference is profound compared with the rear. Also, notice that it's possible to improve rear-brake traction by shifting your weight off the back of the saddle to above the wheel. And of course, it will be clear that using both brakes in combination yields the best result of all.

There's one more point to this drill: Notice that if either wheel skids, you don't stop as quickly. This is because you lose traction. Doing this drill repeatedly helps you recognize what you're shooting for—the point of maximum stopping power that occurs just before the wheels lock up. You'll even feel your tires "chirp," especially in front, and the bike will try to throw you forward. Use a strong rearward weight shift to keep the wheels just this side of skidding.

Braking in Turns

I became painfully aware of the value of the front brake during a recent group ride through the New Mexico desert. About 10 minutes into the ride, I misjudged a series of high speed dips, buried my front wheel in one of them, and sailed over the bars. When I examined my bike, I found I had bent my front rim so badly that it rubbed against the brake pads. I loosened my front brake cable so the brakes did not rub on the bent rim, but I still had no front braking power.

Without my front brake, I repeatedly approached corners with too much speed. Using the rear brake alone required getting my weight further back and initiating braking much earlier. I hadn't realized how dependent I was on my front brake. The rear's stopping power was pitiful in comparison. That ride was a good lesson on maximizing rear wheel braking traction and the superiority of the front brake.

But never forget the following words about grabbing the front brake hard while in a downhill turn: Don't do it. When you hit the front brake while the bike is leaning and gravity is pulling, only bad things can happen. The bike will want to become more upright and take a straighter line. Chances are very good that this is not the reaction you're hoping for. The consequences can be particularly brutal on a side hill where you might plunge over the edge.

Control your speed before you lean, then get off the brakes an instant before you enter the turn. If your speed is still too great, resist the temptation to grab the front brake. This will almost certainly cause the front wheel to wash out, and down you'll go. Instead, keep leaning in and use the rear brake. A rear-wheel skid is more controllable and can even help redirect the bike onto the right line. This is worth practicing, so I'll tell you how.

First, let me emphasize that intentionally skidding on singletrack is a major no-no. It's not trail friendly. It widens and scars the trail, opening the door to damaging erosion. Never skid on singletrack unless it's to save your skin. Even that's a weak excuse. You should control your speed so you don't get into situations that require extreme measures. But mistakes do happen.

Practice this technique on a dirt road where skidding is inconsequential. Pick a certain spot to initiate your turn. Build some speed, get your weight back as I've described, then lean in. Now hit the rear brake hard enough to lock the wheel just for a second and cause it to slide toward the outside of the turn, pivoting the bike. Instantly, you'll be on a tighter line. Countersteer with the front wheel by turning it toward the outside of the turn. This helps you control the amount of rear-wheel slide. Then release the brake before your momentum is lost, and go. Practice left and right turns this way until you feel confident in your ability to induce and control a skid. Usually when a wheel breaks loose, it means loss of control, but in this instance it helps you regain control. Learn not to keep the brake on too long and plunge from too much speed to no speed. Practice will also give you the feel for lever modulation.

A variation is necessary when you're making a faster or tighter turn, especially on a slippery surface. The basic technique is the same, but it helps to take your inside foot off the pedal and use it as an outrigger. I'll tell you about this in chapter 15, High-Speed Turns.

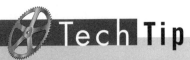

If you're going to use your brakes as hard as I'm recommending, you need maximum leverage and power. Your mountain bike is likely to have one of three braking systems: cantilever, parallel-pull, or disc.

Cantilever. Stopping power is affected most by the height of the straddle cable that connects the two arms. The lower the cable, the farther out the arms will be, and the more power you'll get. Shoot for a 90-degree angle between each arm and the cable. But make sure the cable doesn't hit the tire or reduce mud clearance.

Parallel-pull. This type (also known as direct-pull or by Shimano's brand name, V-Brake) is superior to the cantilever because it's more powerful and reduces the risk of a brake pad sliding up into the tire or down into the spokes. For these reasons, parallel-pull brakes became standard equipment on better bikes in the late 1990s. After the pads are positioned to hit the rim squarely, make adjustments to braking leverage at the levers themselves.

Disc. Unlike the first two types, disc brakes operate at the hub rather than at the rim. This location keeps them cleaner, and their design gives them various mechanical advantages. In fact, they're an offshoot of the brakes found on motorcycles. In my experience, it's the innate quality and design of a given disc brake that produces excellent stopping power, not tweaks that you make after the fact. The difference between a good disc brake and a mediocre one is in the modulation it allows. If it simply works like a light switch (on/off), it's poorly designed. Also, look for a system that doesn't leave pads in continuous contact with the discs.

Lever position. It's best to position the brake levers so your wrists are straight when braking from out of the saddle, as on a fast or technical downhill. Move the levers laterally on the bar until you can easily reach their ends with your index and middle fingers (or even one finger if your hands are strong enough). This creates the most leverage. Fine-tune lever play by turning the cable adjustment barrel. The brake pads should not make contact until the lever is relatively close to the bar, where your hand strength is greatest. However, the wheel should lock up before the lever actually reaches the bar.

Pad selection. Brake pads can wear out in as little as one ride. When you need to replace your pads, you're not limited to original equipment. Several companies make aftermarket pads with compounds designed for specific riding conditions. Whatever you use, frequently check pad condition and replace them sooner rather than later. If pads wear out during a ride, the metal-to-metal contact can ruin your rims.

Sloppy Stops

Braking in wet or muddy conditions can provide some unwanted thrills if you don't think. The main thing to remember is how poorly rim brakes respond in the slop. This is why disc brakes began catching on in the late 1990s and why they look like a lock to become stock equipment on many performance bikes.

If you have discs, braking response won't change throughout the range of environmental conditions. But if you use parallel-pull or cantilever brakes, pad friction against the rim runs the gamut from excellent to awful. To compensate in bad conditions, you need to ride with anticipation and a heightened sense of your bike's position relative to vertical.

On wet, slippery surfaces, you can't lean as far into a turn or brake as hard. The rims are likely to be slick, too, so you need to brake sooner and with more modulation. The pads won't start gripping until gunk is wiped away, then braking power comes on suddenly. If you squeeze the levers hard, the wheels may instantly skid when the pads bite. Combine this with even a little turning action, and you need lots of luck to stay upright. Wheels go away with little provocation in wet conditions.

This risk is something riders face when racing at Mount Snow, Vermont, home to numerous big events over the years. The course is infamous for its wet roots and rocks. On descents, all you can do is point the bike in the right direction, get off the brakes, and hold on. Lines become much more important when a descent is wet. The rear brake is only semi-useful in conditions like these, so you really need to concentrate on finding places where you can safely use the front. The worst thing you can do is be on the front brake when going over a diagonal root. Your wheel will slide right down the thing. You'll be riding the root instead of your bike.

Fly when Dry

Take advantage of good braking conditions by waiting until the last moment to grab the levers, especially in a race when the course is dry. In this way, you'll waste minimal time while still scrubbing off enough speed to get through turns safely.

In sand, brake as little as possible, because it's so easy to lose momentum. The soft surface will slow you very quickly as soon as you stop pedaling, so anticipate this and don't lose even more speed by braking. Adjustments to pedal pressure may be all you need on some sandy courses.

In less mushy stuff—say, powdery dirt with a hard surface underneath—braking technique becomes crucial again. You really have to be careful in downhill turns. If you book through with too much speed, your front wheel will slide in the powder instead of finding traction. This will take you to the outside of the turn—or worse, right off the trail.

If you try to brake in this situation, you can kiss your momentum goodbye. I saw this happen to a rider at the Iron Horse Classic in Durango, Colorado. This guy was good enough to win pro cross-country races, but on this dusty course he made the same mistake on every downhill turn. Most of them were a bit off-camber, and so the ground's sloping to the outside made them even more difficult. He was on the front brake going in, causing his wheel to plow straight through the turn's apex instead of following its radius. After losing momentum in the soft stuff beside the trail, he pedaled up to speed—then did it all over again at the next opportunity. Instead, he should have committed to a line, adjusted his speed on the approach, released the brakes, and rolled through the turn. Front-wheel braking never works in turns with a loose surface.

8 Riding with Others

Boost Your Fun, Safety, and Learning Curve

Legend has it that my co-author, Ed Pavelka, bought the first mountain bike sold in Vermont. This was in early 1982. It was a Specialized Stumpjumper, the first mountain bike to be mass-produced. He still owns this relic. It's now preserved like a museum piece.

Back then, Ed was a road rider and trail runner. Where he lived in southern Vermont, there were miles of abandoned logging roads and forest trails starting at his back door. When a knee injury made it risky to continue running, he figured that his days in the woods might be over. It wasn't a happy thought. Then, like the answer to a prayer, that Stumpjumper appeared in one of Vermont's classic little bike stores, the West Hill Shop in Putney. Suddenly, the trails were open again.

Ed rode his Stumpjumper for the next couple of years, but he always rode alone. No rider near him had a mountain bike yet. He learned how to ride by trial and error, figuring out for himself many of the moves described in this book—or at least as many as he could imagine. One of his favorite trails was a loop that took about 45 minutes to ride. It included nearly every obstacle—rocks, roots, ruts, logs, ledges, ditches, slippery climbs, and even a pond with an old beaver dam that he could ride across (sometimes). He made a game of trying to complete the entire loop without putting a foot down. He began to succeed more often than not. He thought he must have been pretty good.

Then Ed visited Crested Butte, Colorado, to ride at one of the first Fat Tire Bike Weeks. Guys rode around him. Women dropped him. Elderly hikers asked him to please get out of their way. It was almost like he'd never been on a mountain bike before. He stumbled and stalled where other riders made it look easy. He realized that all of his solo riding back home had done very little to teach him the skills and speed that other riders were developing. He learned as much during one week with good riders on Rocky Mountain singletrack as he had in two seasons of riding alone.

Two or More Is Better Than One

Sure, it's fine to ride solo occasionally to clear your head or work on a specific skill. The key word is "occasionally." In my experience, there's no faster way to get good than by riding with others—especially if they are a bit better than you. By following the line of a good rider and watching him handle obstacles, your sense of what is possible on a mountain bike will expand. In a similar way, an instructional video will broaden your horizons. I'm partial to "Ned Overend's Performance Mountain Biking," which I made for Performance Video and Instruction. To order the video, write to 550 Riverbend, Durango, CO 81301; or call (888) 259-5805.

One of my best friends in Durango is Daryl Price, who was a top pro for many years. We often trained together, and this made both of us better.

It can get competitive when riding with friends, and that's good. By pushing each other, you'll improve your fitness and bike-handling skills faster than by always riding solo.

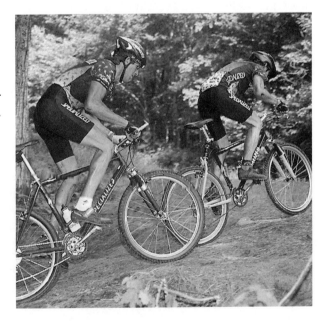

Often, our rides became impromptu races. I would lead for awhile and try to drop him, then he would lead and try to bury me. We would get on long climbs and ramp up the pace, seeing who would blow first. His strengths improved my weaknesses, and vice versa. These rides were not only effective but they were also fun because we didn't let them get dangerous. We used our heads. Part of learning is discovering where the edge is and not riding over it. If you throw yourself on the ground regularly, you and your equipment are going to be laid up too often to improve.

Pro racer John Tomac taught me to be a better descender. He didn't do it on purpose, though. Because John was a superior downhiller when we started racing against each other, I got many chances to watch him from behind. I improved by copying his lines and his moves. My goal was to stay with him farther down each hill. He made me push the envelope. It's great how well this worked. The longer I was able to hang with John, the more I learned, and the more my confidence grew. And, of course, the less advantage he had.

Conversely, think about what happens when you ride downhill alone. You have no one to draw you out. There's no example to watch, no one to keep up with, no challenge. The result is that you rarely ride at your limit or slightly beyond—the point at which real learning takes place. You may be timid because there's no one to help you if you crash. This is actually smart thinking. You don't want to be hurt in the woods alone. But it's also a big drawback of riding solo.

Plenty of Space

When riding singletrack behind a good rider, you want to be close enough to see how he takes a turn, unweights over obstacles, and makes other moves. But don't get too close. You must leave a safety margin. If he happens to wad it up, you need enough time and space to avoid hitting him. Also, by hanging back, you give him some breathing room. When you're right on a guy's rear wheel, he feels the pressure and may ride more recklessly to keep his speed. His concentration is split between what is behind and what is ahead—a recipe for mistakes.

There's another problem if you're too close. Think about what happens if the guy in front suddenly swerves to avoid a rock or stump. If you can't see several feet of open ground between his rear wheel and your front wheel, you're on top of the obstacle before you have time to avoid it. Don't get so caught up in watching him that you fail to watch out for yourself. The faster

Ned's KNOWLEDGE

One fun benefit of riding with friends is trying their bikes. For example, my good friend Daryl Price and I have almost identical seat heights. This makes it easy to swap bikes for part of a ride to sample different equipment. One year, his bike had Shimano components, a Rock Shox fork, and Continental tires, while I was riding Grip Shift, Manitou, and Specialized. It's interesting to check out competing products.

Trade bikes when you're on group rides. You may discover equipment or a bike setup that suits you better. The next time you need to replace or upgrade a part, you'll have the experience to make a smarter choice.

you're going, the more focus you must have on your own situation. When the pace is more casual, you can pay more attention to how the other guy is handling the trail.

Even when riding side by side on a dirt road, leave room for error. Keep in mind that any unpaved surface is likely to be rough and provide less-than-perfect traction. Each of you watches for rocks, ruts, holes, or soft spots. Evasive swerves can clang you together. For the same reason, obey the roadie rule that says never overlap wheels when riding behind someone. If your front wheel is up beside the other guy's rear wheel and he swerves unexpectedly, the contact is very likely to knock you down.

One Big Game

In Durango, there's a difficult climb through a rough, rocky technical section. It's known simply as the Ridge. To ride through it, you have to ratchet the pedals to keep them from hitting the rocks. It's a real challenge. If I don't make it without putting a foot down, that's unacceptable. I go back down and try it again. When I'm riding with friends, this turns into a contest. We go one at a time to see who can make it. The encouragement and camaraderie draws out the best in everyone.

In a similar way, I preride each race course with a teammate so we can try different lines through tough sections. I've done this many times with my friend and fellow racer Steve Tilford. Maybe he sees a line that I don't. Maybe we're both stumped. By talking it over and trying different gears and lines, we're more likely to find a solution together than if we were on our own. This is especially true at a technical course like Vermont's Mount Snow. You can burn lots of energy trying to learn the toughest sections just before a race, so it really helps to have two brains working.

Enough Fun for Everyone

Another advantage of riding with other people is that you're sharing experiences. Mountain biking is a ton of fun. Riding great singletrack is one of those things in life that are impossible to describe adequately to someone who hasn't done them. The joy of carving a twisty section, the beauty of an unexpected overlook, or the satisfaction of cleaning a technical climb seems to last forever when you share these memorable moments with other riders. Recollections flood in whenever someone asks, "Remember that time. . . ?" How many solo experiences can you recall that you thought you'd never forget?

There's also an important safety factor. This is especially true on epic rides that take you into the backcountry, far from help. When you ride with friends, an injury or mechanical breakdown doesn't leave you stranded. You have people to get you going again or get you help. But auger in alone, and you could wind up in a desperate situation. Before any backcountry ride, always tell a responsible person where you're headed and what time you expect to be back, just in case.

Local Talent

I travel a lot, so I'm frequently in a new place without a clue about where to go for a ride. Sometimes, you'll find yourself in this situation, too, whether you've packed your mountain bike or road bike. Call or visit the local bicycle shops and ask about a club ride. Maybe you can pick up a club newsletter or local recreation paper that lists cycling activities. Even if nothing organized is going on, chances are good that you'll find a rider or two who will be happy to take you out.

What's interesting about these rides is how spirited they often become. Maybe it's because the local riders want to see how they compare to the stranger in town, or perhaps they just want to stick up for the talent in their club. Either way, I love the result—they push me and I get fitness from the ride. This is so much better than going out alone on the local bike route. It's just one more advantage of riding with others.

9 Trail Friendliness

Ride Like Our Sport
Depends on You—Because It Does

This book's main goal is to help you ride trails with skill and control. The result is more fun on your bike, but it goes even further than that. You'll also be a safer rider, able to negotiate challenging singletrack with less risk of crashes and damage to yourself, other trail users, and even the trail itself. To ride safely, you need to build technique before building speed.

As a mountain biker, you're the fastest nonmotorized person on any trail. Your speed in most situations is much greater than that of the other two groups of trail users whom you're likely to encounter—pedestrians (hikers, backpackers, and runners) and equestrians (horseback riders). It's easy to imagine the potential dangers on narrow trails with blind turns.

In the early years of mountain biking, there were enough conflicts with other trail users to result in some prime singletrack being closed to cyclists. Remember, we are the newcomers. Pedestrians and equestrians have had trails all to themselves for centuries, and they also have well-established local and national organizations to influence trail-use policy. We mountain bikers immediately found ourselves on the defensive, losing ground (literally) in the fight to legally ride great singletrack around the country. In response, riders began forming local trail-access groups. The most active were in California, where the mountain bike was invented, and riders were soon in conflict with traditional trail users.

Well, as usual, trends from the West Coast moved across the nation. Mountain bikers nearly everywhere were being banned from trails. Local groups started fighting back, but they were underpowered compared to those trying to keep bikes away. In 1988, the International Mountain Bicycling Association (IMBA) was founded to give the sport a unified national voice in access issues. Since then, IMBA has turned the tide. It has given mountain bikers a respected position in the family of U.S. trail users, and it's striving to make an equal impact worldwide.

IMBA's basic individual membership is $20 per year. Five higher levels of support are offered. For information, contact IMBA at P.O. Box 7578, Boulder, CO 80306-7578, or visit the Web site at www.imba.com.

Our Responsibilities

As trail riders, it's imperative that we support IMBA and our local mountain bike access groups. If we don't help with our membership dollars and volunteer labor, who will preserve our access to singletrack, maintain these trails, and build new ones? The answer is easy: no one. It's up to each of us.

There's a second component, too. We need to ride responsibly in terms of environmental impact, not just human impact. Taking machines into the backcountry was enough to initially create ill feelings among pedestrians and equestrians. The fact that our bikes are capable of damaging trails has been used since day one in their attempt to restrict us from singletrack. But it's not the bike that's the problem, it's how the bike is ridden. (It's the same for hiking boots, if you think about it. Put them on a pair of reckless feet, and damage may follow.) Avoid shortcuts across turns, and you won't create erosion paths that gash trails. For the same reason, don't skid your wheels or ride when the trail is muddy. All these things produce ruts that water can follow. Just as important, avoid riding off the trail. Especially in the desert, your tires can leave scars that last for years.

Be respectful of private property. Trespassing is illegal and it gives mountain bikers a bad image. Always ride in control, but especially when you have a limited sight distance. Even if your speed is well within your capabilities, you need to respect the fact that you can still scare the heck out of pedestrians who don't realize how quickly a mountain bike can stop. I see this happen all the time. There's plenty of room for riders to react, but pedestrians who suddenly see them coming dive off the trail. The pedestrians aren't really in danger, but they don't realize this until too late.

Passing others is the most important part of trail relationships, according

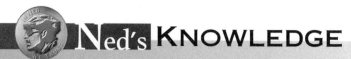

Ned's KNOWLEDGE

When each of us rides by the six principles of the International Mountain Bicycling Association, we go a long way toward protecting the privilege of using public trails. Do your part to make mountain biking a safe and enjoyable experience for every trail user—pedestrians, equestrians, and fellow mountain bikers.

1. Ride on open trails only.
2. Leave no trace.
3. Control your bicycle.
4. Always yield trail.
5. Never spook animals.
6. Plan ahead.

to my friend Tim Blumenthal, the executive director of IMBA and a former editor at *Bicycling* and *Mountain Bike* magazines. "It's what causes other trail users to feel positive or negative about mountain bikers," he explains. When you encounter pedestrians, follow IMBA's simple advice: (1) slow down, (2) establish communication, (3) be prepared to stop, (4) pass safely.

It's certainly easier for a hiker to step aside than it is for a rider to stop and let a hiker walk past. But it's still the rider's responsibility to yield, so be ready in case you need to. When a pedestrian does move over to let you pass, thank him. Always be cordial. After all, a hiker, backpacker, or runner is out there for the same positive reasons you are. No one's day should be ruined by an unpleasant encounter.

Horse Sense

Equestrians are a whole different situation. Horses are very skittish around bikes. This is certainly true in Colorado and other places where outfitters lead hunting parties in the fall. Most pack horses have been out to pasture all summer. They're usually nervous about the change in their environment. There they are on a tight trail, and along you come on your mountain bike. It can be a real hassle to get past. The horses often will turn in circles and make life hard for the people trying to control them.

Always yield to equestrians. I'm talking 100 percent of the time. When approaching from the front, stop and move as far off the trail as practical. There's usually less chance that a horse will freak if it sees you coming, as opposed to unexpectedly hearing you coming from behind. When you approach from the front, its rider will see you, too, and be ready for any frightened reaction. When you come from the back, the horse will probably hear you before the rider does and may bolt before the rider has any reason to expect a problem.

Horses are much more jumpy about strange and potentially dangerous sounds—the snap of a shifter, pedal, or brake lever—than they are about a human voice, which they usually associate with kindness or food. So if you come up from behind and your presence is unnoticed, say something before making any other noise. Don't yell, just use a friendly tone and enough volume to be heard. The rider will get the message at the same time that the horse does, so there's less chance of a problem. When approaching from either direction, stop until the rider has control. Wait till he indicates how he'd like the pass to be made.

A Louder Voice

We can't just take from our sport. We must give something back. Each of us needs to stand up for mountain biking and be counted.

The more people who have paid for memberships to IMBA, the more clout IMBA will have when working for our sport in Washington, D.C., and with the field offices of the federal land agencies—the National Park Service, U.S. Forest Service, and Bureau of Land Management. It's essential for each of us to be on IMBA's rolls in the national effort. As of 1998, IMBA had 13,000 dues-paying members in all 50 states and 30 countries, plus 350 member clubs that had a total of 70,000 members. That's pretty impressive after just 10 years of existence, but it's still only a fraction of the millions of people who ride mountain bikes.

Just as important are the hundreds of local trails organizations around the country. To find out if there is one in your area, ask at your local bike club or shop, or contact IMBA. Then join. The modest dues are vital for protecting trail access and even expanding off-road cycling opportunities. Most groups have newsletters or Web sites to keep riders abreast of regional issues affecting the sport.

You'll most likely be offered the chance to participate in a trail-maintenance day. This is not just a way to repair the land, it's a way to build community relations. It shows that mountain bikers are more than the nose rings, spiked hair, and big air that are portrayed in TV commercials. It shows that we're responsible people who are willing to work for the good of the environment that we use.

Political Clout

When it comes to local politics, an organized mountain bike group proves that there is a constituency of cyclists. This makes it more likely that incumbents and candidates will pay attention to access issues. A group also provides a cohesive voice in dealings with other trail-use associations. Without this, we may not be heard and conflicts won't be resolved fairly.

I saw the benefits firsthand in Durango, Colorado, when a problem arose with some outfitters and their pack horses. They complained to the Forest Service that mountain bikers were scaring the horses, which created a dangerous situation for people in the hunting parties. The outfitters wanted a certain trail closed to cyclists. This created two problems. First, lots of Durango riders liked using the trail. Second, if we lost that trail, which one would be next?

Durango has a well-established organization called Trails 2000. Its membership includes not just mountain bikers but also runners, hikers, and even some equestrians. We scheduled a meeting to discuss the issue. Attending were the outfitters and representatives from the Forest Service and Bureau of Land Management. By discussing issues, we realized we could appreciate each other's situation. The mountain bikers admitted there were some irresponsible riders who were doing things that scared the horses. The outfitters admitted that some of the horses had been out to pasture for months and weren't used to walking the trails. It wasn't a one-sided problem.

After we reached this understanding, it was easy to find a solution that was much less severe than trail closure. Trails 2000 agreed to put signs in bike shops and at the trailhead to warn riders that they were likely to encounter horses during the autumn. Some riders decided to avoid the trail at this time of year, and those who continued to ride were more careful. Peer pressure had something to do with it. We knew that if trouble persisted, we would lose the trail. No one wanted to be responsible for that.

Similar problems are being resolved every week around the country. In many places, the original bike-unfriendly trail policy of "closed unless open" has been reversed, thanks to the work of IMBA and local access groups. We've earned a fair shake, but our access will never be secure unless we support the organizations that protect it.

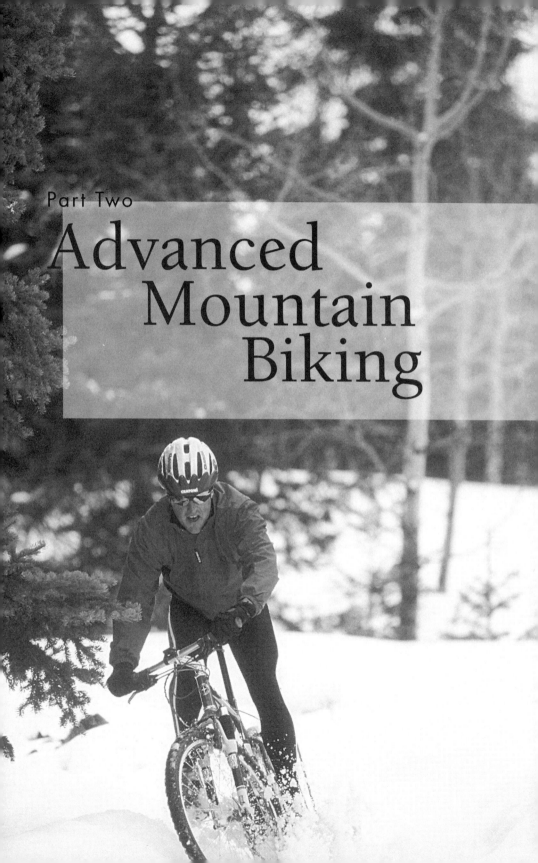

Part Two

Advanced Mountain Biking

10 Suspension

Ways to Make Trails Less Shocking

You're reading this book because you'd like to widen the range of technical terrain that you can ride well. Let me tell you the easiest way to improve. Use suspension. Whether it's provided by your body or the bike, suspension buffers the jitters and jolts that reduce control and increase fatigue. It's the area in which there have been the greatest technological advancements, and you can safely bet that many more will come.

I wasn't always quite so optimistic. The first time I rode a bike with a suspension fork, I remember thinking, "This thing will never work." Now, as I write this barely a decade later, it's hard to find a mountain bike without front suspension. Most racers haven't been on a rigid fork in years. And despite my initial misgivings, the bike I now ride most often is a dualie—it has rear suspension as well as front. I'm positive we'll see dual suspension capture the mountain bike market, and for good reason. It helps every rider perform better.

The Evolution

Suspension does for the rider what the rider once had to do for himself—absorb the body-rattling shocks of riding over rough ground. On rigid mountain bikes, this was accomplished with flexed elbows and knees. A rider protected himself from impacts by crouching off the saddle in the attack position, letting the bike buck beneath him. If he didn't get off the saddle, he got pounded. Motorcycle-like suspension forks were a logical first solution, being fairly simple to adapt to bicycles. By buffering front-wheel impacts, they made it possible to go faster with more control. A rider's hands, arms, and shoulders liked the extra up-front comfort, too.

But the job wasn't finished. Bikes with no rear suspension are known as hardtails, and you know what this implies. It wasn't long before attention turned to the rear wheel. After all, a rider's butt is right above it. The pounding can be severe. It's also easy to imagine how sparing riders' legs from jolts can leave them fresher to help them pedal stronger.

Unlike the development of the shock-absorbing fork, though, the evolution of rear suspension has been all over the drawing board. There has been very little agreement among engineers as to what makes the most effective system, but each year the bikes perform better. Once bike weight fell to less than 25 pounds, there was no downside to riding a well-designed dualie. Even ounce-conscious racers realize that on many courses, the benefits of dual suspension overcome a slight weight penalty. This is certainly true when there's lots of rough downhill.

Dual suspension will absolutely increase the variety of technical terrain you can ride, even if your skill level remains constant. Suspension is forgiving. It takes up slack in your technique. It keeps your tires on the ground so you have better steering control and braking traction. You can climb

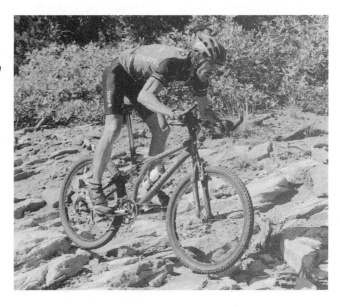

This is the type of terrain in which dual suspension really pays off. A dualie's ability to suck up jolts for you reduces fatigue while increasing comfort. You can often remain in the saddle on rough stuff.

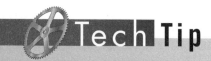

Every suspension fork and rear-suspension system comes with instructions on how to tune it for best performance. Read this material and learn what those knobs are for. Then use them. Too many riders don't maximize their bikes' shock-absorbing ability by adjusting the suspensions for their weight and riding surface.

The adjustments aren't difficult. *Spring rate* determines how much of the suspension's range of motion is used (by determining the amount of force required to compress the suspension). Set the *preload* so your system is responsive to small hits and occasionally bottoms out on the biggest ones. This will give you the full range of movement in typical terrain. Depending on your suspension, spring rate is adjustable via air, elastomers, or a metal coil. The first is easy to adjust with a pump, while the other two require part changes.

Damping is the other factor in suspension setup. There are two types in each suspension, compression and rebound, which are usually controlled by a plunger running through oil. Damping lets you tune the shock's reaction to a bump. You want the shock to return to its original position and be prepared for the next hit, but not recoil so fast that it causes the bike to bounce.

It's best to experiment. Generally, if you want a more efficient setup (stiffer suspension action) you need to run a little higher spring rate or higher preload. This will reduce pedaling-induced suspension movement on the flatter, smoother sections of a trail. But it may also reduce the shock's ability to soak up little bumps. Keep adjusting and testing to find the efficiency-to-plushness ratio that suits your terrain and riding style.

Once you have the hang of your system, you'll feel confident to customize the settings for the terrain of a particular ride. I do this a lot. For instance, if I'm racing on a fairly smooth course, I crank up the preload and increase the compression and rebound damping. I want the suspension to be less active. If it's a rough course, I back off the preload and lighten the damping. On most suspension systems, these adjustments are easy to make using external knobs, if you know the direction and amount to turn them. Follow the directions in the owner's manual.

One final tip: Don't set it and forget it. Eventually, your suspension system will begin to respond differently for various reasons, such as loss of air pressure or the oil becoming contaminated with dust. Wear occurs to springs, elastomers, pivots, and bushings—just think of all the abuse your bike goes through. The key to reliable and predictable performance is to service your suspension according to the owner's manual.

steeper grades with some rear suspensions because they leverage the rear wheel into the ground, producing more tire bite. And, of course, like a down-hill racer, you can descend at greater speed without sacrificing control. This is the advantage that draws many riders to dual suspension in the first place.

In cross-country races, the benefits of a dualie always become apparent in the last hour. You feel fresher than the guys on hardtails if it's a rough course. Your chances of picking them off and moving up in the standings are greater. This freshness factor is easy to understand when you consider the rigors of pedaling hard on choppy ground. Each bump you hit adds to stress on your muscles. When you reduce this stress with dual suspension, you feel less fatigue in the race and less soreness the next day. The same goes when you train on a dualie instead of on a hardtail, and that's why I do it.

Body Suspension

Even on a dualie, you need to make use of your body's shock-absorbing system. Although mechanical suspension lets you be more subtle in using your body as suspension, your arms and legs are still essential.

It all comes back to riding relaxed. Have a firm grip on the handlebar but let your body be supple. Be fluid in your movements, like a shock absorber that has oil damping. The oil is in your wrists, elbows, and shoulders as well as in your ankles, knees, and hips. Prevent tenseness in these joints so they can flex to reduce the shock that reaches your torso and head.

Let's say you're riding over a rough, slightly downhill section. The goal here is to let your bike float under you with the wheels flowing along the contour of the ground. You're in the attack position with the crankarms horizontal and your butt back, just above the saddle. Your arms and legs move up, down, back, and forward, but your head barely bobs at all. Now you can focus on picking your line and holding it, helped by the fact that the tires are not bouncing off the ground.

Use the same posture if you have to pedal through rough stuff. Unless you're on a dualie, you can't sit, so find a rhythm by timing your pedal strokes with the undulations. Pedal in circles with supple legs and hips. Crouch more toward the front, as opposed to when you're just coasting. Your knees shouldn't straighten. In fact, they may have even more bend than when you're sitting.

During most seated pedaling, you can have your body weight fully on the saddle. On rougher sections, use pedaling pressure to elevate your butt slightly. It's easier to do this if you give your legs more resistance by using a slightly bigger gear. Relax and sit when the trail smoothes out.

Arm action is pretty consistent through all this. Have a firm grip for control, but maintain loose wrists, elbows, and shoulders to absorb the chop. One situation that requires a more extreme movement is what I call sucking it up. This happens when you come to a hump across the trail. As your front wheel rolls up onto it, pull back so the bar comes almost to your chest. Then extend your arms, pushing down as you go over the top. This is like doing a pushup on the bike, or an exaggerated rowing motion. It makes the bike follow the contour of the ground for maximum control, instead of launching into the air.

Doing a Dualie

Dual suspension may conjure up visions of screaming downhills and launches over wheel-swallowing ditches, but it's a misconception to think that it's meant only for extreme terrain. Dual suspension works well for all conditions—if you know how to use it.

The shocks on a dualie are usually set up for a 160- to 190-pound rider. Adjusting preload (initial spring tension) will help tailor the ride to your weight. But if you're a featherweight or a Clydesdale, the springs may need to be replaced. Most suspension makers offer aftermarket spring-tweaking kits (stiffer or softer metal coils or elastomers).

The first time I raced on dual suspension was in 1997 at the Vail, Colorado, World Cup. Now, I use a dualie so much that my hardtail is gathering dust. It's the same for more and more riders, but I notice that many of them aren't making full use of dual suspension's advantages. Instead, they're riding with their hardtail habits. Here's how to break free.

Let the bike do the work. On climbs, dual suspension is most effective when you stay seated and let it absorb rough terrain. Climbing in the saddle is more efficient because you aren't supporting your body weight—all your energy goes into ascending the hill. A dualie makes seated climbing more comfortable because the rear wheel follows the contours of the terrain and the saddle doesn't bash your crotch.

Pedal in circles. Riders who stomp the pedals aren't good candidates for dualies. But if you practice turning a full, smooth circle, you'll eliminate most of the energy-sapping bounce associated with dual suspension.

Save your energy. Dual suspension really comes into its own on climbs with little ledges, logs, or roots. On a hardtail, you have to pull up on the front end, then shift your weight forward to get the rear wheel over these obstacles. This movement uses extra energy. Instead, stay seated on a dualie and simply ride across. Even if you must stand, avoid elevating the front wheel or shifting your weight more than necessary.

Don't always get air. Because I rode a hardtail for so long, it was difficult for me to break the habit of unweighting over or steering around rocks on descents. Dual suspension reduces the need to unweight over bumps. Focus on riding right over the small stuff rather than hopping over it; it's less fatiguing.

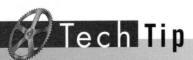

Tech Tip

If you're riding a bike with front suspesnsion and aren't ready to spring for a dual-suspension bike just yet, there's an easy and relatively cheap way to get rear suspension: Install a shock-absorbing seatpost. There are two basic types.

The simpler design looks much like a regular seatpost. It contains elastomers or a spring and slides up and down in line with the bike's bottom bracket. This works, but it has the drawback of changing your seat height as you ride over bumps that are big enough to activate the post. Also, because your weight isn't always centered on the saddle, the forces applied to the post aren't always in line with its movement. This increases friction and wear, possibly resulting in looseness over time.

The other type is more complex, which makes it heavier and more costly. In my experience, though, it also works better. Atop this post is a parallelogram, a four-bar linkage that absorbs bumps by moving horizontally more than vertically. It makes sort of an arc relative to the bottom bracket. This keeps the seat's height quite constant, though it does slightly vary its distance to the handlebar.

A shock post isn't as effective as an integrated rear suspension, but it's a good addition to any hardtail. It lets you stay seated longer on rough terrain. Anytime you're in the saddle, you're more efficient because you're not using muscles to support your weight. Of course, when you stand, a shock post has no effect, so on bumpy downhills you definitely miss the benefits of active rear-wheel suspension. A post also can't improve traction on out-of-saddle climbs by leveraging your rear wheel into the ground. But it does have the advantage of mechanical simplicity and pedaling efficiency, especially when you're standing on smooth climbs.

I put a suspension seatpost on my wife's bike. It made a ton of difference to her enjoyment because she doesn't ride enough to develop great technique. Now she no longer fears being pounded by the saddle.

Adjust the suspension to get full travel only on the biggest hits. You don't want to bottom out very often. But if you never bottom out, you aren't benefiting from the suspension's full range. To see how much travel you're getting, put one zip-tie around a fork leg and another around the rear shock, then note how far they move during a ride. Measure the distance and compare it to the manufacturer's specifications.

Ratchet the pedals. Dual suspension tempts you to pedal through anything, so be careful not to catch a pedal on a rock or the high side of a trail. Realize that when the suspension is compressed, the bottom bracket is lower, leaving less clearance between the pedals and the ground. Some of my worst crashes have been from bashing a pedal. The bike jumps to one side and down you go. Ratchet through tricky sections by taking a partial stroke, backpedaling for a partial stroke, then taking another partial stroke. Or just coast with the crankarms parallel to the ground if you have enough momentum.

Go wide in the turns. Dual suspension's generous travel means you can push the bike down with the outside pedal and carve turns like a skier. But watch out—long-travel forks make the head-tube angle steepen when the fork is compressed, quickening the steering response. If you should brake hard on a steep downhill switchback, the fork will dive and the turning radius could suddenly be too tight. Compensate by taking a wider line. Better yet, slow to the correct speed before you start turning.

Beware the "Yee-hah!" factor. Dual suspension lets you go faster even if you don't have great technique. That's fine as long as you realize that if you do fall, it will hurt a lot more. Don't get in over your head.

Dualing for Dollars

Shopping for a dual-suspension bike can be almost as tough as forecasting the marketplace. What can I tell you about current dualies that will still be relevant when you're reading this a year or more later? Technology is moving like a downhill racer—fast and progressive, but still hitting some bumps along the way. There's little use discussing the suspension features of specific bike models, when new and improved designs are continuously being introduced.

Things seem to be settling down in one respect, however. Most dualies can be categorized as one of three types, each with a distinct personality. One is the so-called freeride or big-hit or downhill bike. I think of it more as a chairlift bike. This is a relatively high-price model that weighs close to

71

30 pounds because it's loaded with suspension—at least 5 inches in back and 4 or more inches in front, with a hefty triple-crown fork to control the motion. You can ride these bikes in most terrain, but they are really tough to pedal uphill because of their weight and suspension action. They're popular at ski areas, where riders can take them on chairlifts to the top then enjoy the plush ride to the bottom.

Next is the category that my sponsor, Specialized, terms enduro. These dualies have 4 or 5 inches of rear travel with about 3 inches of fork travel. This results in a bike that's not quite as absorbent as a freeride bike, but it's several pounds lighter and more efficient. It's designed for general recreation but really shines on rough trails and during epic rides that venture into a wide range of terrain.

I think of the third category as the sports-car category. It can be termed cross-country or XC. This is the dualie for those who want all-around performance. Suspension travel is reduced to about 3 inches in both front and rear to save weight and improve pedaling efficiency. Less travel also allows a lower bottom bracket, which lowers the center of gravity—an important advantage for cornering. And there's less change in steering geometry as the suspension activates, a benefit when riding through bumpy turns. Because air shocks are often used, XC bikes are the lightest of the dualies, weighing in at around 23 pounds. All of these attributes make them the right choice for racing. Their ride may not be as plush as that of the bikes in the other two categories, but less energy is lost to suspension movement. To riders who think more travel means a faster bike, remember that you have to ride to the top of the hill before you get to descend. An XC dualie goes up quicker, and it isn't that much slower going down.

When you go shopping, you'll find numerous bikes in each category using a variety of front and rear suspensions. The best way to choose is by taking test-rides to see what meets your needs and riding style. Every design has pluses and minuses. For example, a suspension system that becomes less active when you stand helps you climb more efficiently. But it also isn't as active when you're standing on descents, which is the most common riding position when the ground is rough.

When you're ready to buy, read reviews of the latest systems in bike magazines, read manufacturers' literature, talk with local riders and shop mechanics, and take those test-rides. Remember, for all-around cross-country riding and racing, you want to be on suspension that strikes a balance between active and efficient.

11 Momentum

Keep Big Mo Working for You

It's great to be on singletrack when everything is clicking. You brake just enough. You hit the right gear so you don't stall coming out of turns. You ride over obstacles like they are not even there. Everything just flows.

There's a word for what this produces, and the word is "momentum." So much of riding is about preserving the drive and force that a rider's energy imparts to the bike. Braking, turning, climbing, negotiating obstacles . . . everything. An essential ingredient is how shock is absorbed with flexed arms and legs and the bike's suspension. This is what keeps a rider moving forward instead of being bounced upward or backward. A good rider is always trying to milk the terrain for maximum momentum. It's a skill that can continually be improved.

Load and Release

Juli Furtado, one of mountain biking's most dominant racers, often draws an interesting parallel to downhill skiing, another sport in which she excelled. As Juli notes, when you carve a turn, you load the skis. They're a lot like springs. You weight them, then let this energy release as you come out of the turn. The skis actually give energy back to you. On a mountain bike, you accentuate momentum by using your equipment in a similar way.

73

Here's an example. Imagine that you're on a slight downhill. The turns are coming up so quickly that you don't even have time to pedal between them. Each turn has a slight berm, giving the trail a concave shape. You push the bike into this berm as you coil your body like a spring storing energy. It's a subtle movement. As you exit the turn, you extend your arms and legs in an upward motion. You're loading and unloading—actually making the bike surge forward a bit each time. Meanwhile, the guy in front of you is using typical technique—sitting or standing statically, steering instead of carving. You catch him in no time, and the difference is that you're maximizing your momentum.

To ride like this takes a combination of finesse and relaxation. Confidence is part of the formula, too. A great example was Juli's performance at the World Downhill Championship in Bromont, Canada. The course was technical—rough and muddy. Juli, although primarily a cross-country racer

Maximize your momentum by weighting and unweighting through turns. As you enter, push the bike down into the berm while you coil your body like a spring to store energy (top). Then as you exit, extend your arms and legs (bottom). This upward motion makes the bike surge forward—free speed simply by using your body weight in harmony with the terrain.

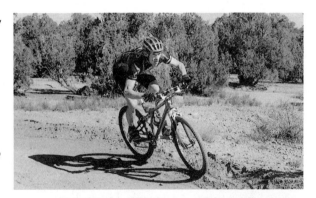

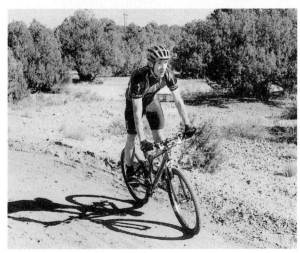

at the time, was competing against powerful women who had prepared specifically for this downhill. They'd done lots of weight training and sprint work. But Juli had a more important advantage. She'd learned how to read terrain as a skier. She maximized her momentum not with brute power but with finesse, choosing the ideal line so she could brake less and preserve her speed through turns. The result was another world championship for her collection.

Juli's victory also illustrates the importance of good vision. This enables you to recognize effective momentum-saving moves. Keep scanning between the trail horizon and your wheel. Choose your immediate line, then look beyond to the next move—farther ahead the faster you're going. The better you read the trail, the more momentum you can keep. But all it takes to kill ol' mo is one moment of unnecessary hesitation. Consider your safety, of course, but don't be too reluctant to commit and go for it.

Better Shifting

Shifting gears fluidly is a major key to momentum, especially on climbs. When gravity is robbing your speed, the correct technique is to shift into each lower gear just before you actually need to. This gives you a more consistent pedaling cadence and moves the chain before it becomes loaded with pedaling pressure. In fact, if you try to downshift the front derailleur when you're pushing hard on the pedals, the derailleur probably won't shift at all. Its spring is not strong enough to derail a tight chain and drop it onto the smaller ring.

If you fail to anticipate and need to downshift when you're already pedaling hard, first surge with several even stronger strokes. This bit of extra speed lets you take pressure off the pedals for half a revolution just as you make the shift. It helps you keep momentum until you can reapply power.

When you do it right—hit timely shifts to keep your legs fluid—you can make the most of your momentum. You'll be flying while others are disappearing behind you. I recently had a good experience like this in a race. The course had a paved downhill where I could tuck tight and coast faster than I could pedal. Then it went right into a dirt climb. I hit the transition and started pedaling my biggest gear as soon as my legs could feel resistance. Then, I progressively downshifted through the cogs and got onto the middle chainring while the chain was still free to move. Meanwhile, other guys were coasting right up to the point where they needed to downshift to

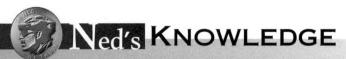

Ned's KNOWLEDGE

You need to be riding a mountain bike to shift it, right? Wrong.

Let's say you're in a race and get bogged down in the wrong gear or someone falls in front of you. You jump off, but now you can't get back on to start riding until the bike is in a lower gear.

You could stop to lift up the rear of the bike, hand pedal, and make the shifts. But here's a better way: Run with the bike. As you're pushing it, move either shifter to a lower gear, then reach down and turn the crankarm with your hand. Keep doing this until the bike is in the right gear for a place where you can remount and begin riding.

I must have done this a hundred times in my racing career. It saves momentum because you never stop moving.

the middle ring before they could pedal. My momentum was so much greater that I could pass four or five of them like they were doing a track-stand. That's what maxing mo is all about.

No More Chainsuck

When you make front downshifts before the chain is loaded with your pedaling pressure, another good thing happens: You reduce the risk of chainsuck. This major mo killer is one of the most frustrating mechanical problems in mountain biking.

Nothing will stop you faster than getting your chain sucked up and jammed tight between the crankset and chainstay. It's easier to avoid if you understand why it happens. The chain is made of steel, a much harder material than the aluminum used in chainrings. When you drop the chain from the middle to the small ring under pressure, it digs into the middle ring and sticks. As the pedal stroke continues, the chain gets pulled up—sucked—and wedged against the chainstay, stopping the crankset cold. Muddy conditions make the chain even more likely to stick.

There are devices that can be bolted to the frame to keep the chain from becoming jammed, but they haven't caught on. I tried one on a bike that was giving me problems. Its position had to be precise and very close to the chainrings, so I found it kind of unworkable. I decided that it's better to prevent chainsuck with good technique and maintenance. Technique was just discussed—anticipate front downshifts so you can make them before putting heavy pressure on the chain.

As for maintenance, keep the chain in good condition. When it's loaded with mud or sand, it's not going to slide off one ring and onto another very well. The same goes when chainring teeth are damaged. Use a file or emery cloth to smooth away nicks, burrs, or other irregularities. Sometimes you'll even find the tops of teeth flattened or hooked because of contact with a rock. Once a tooth is damaged, the chain is likely to stick there again and again.

Three mechanical problems result from chainsuck. First, as you can imagine, it does a number on the chainstay, gouging and scarring it badly. The chain can saw right through an aluminum stay or shred carbon fiber. Second, a chainring can be bent or its teeth can be deformed. The result will be shifting problems and an increased risk of even more chainsuck. Third, it's likely to put a twist in your chain. It could even cause some rivets to pull through. You'll get lousy shifting, drivetrain skipping, or worse—damage from chainsuck is probably the leading cause of broken chains. Often, the chain won't come apart immediately, waiting instead for a time you can least afford to be sidelined—like in a race.

If you stop pedaling the instant you sense the chain being jammed, you can prevent a lot of this damage. Sometimes a quick backpedal will free the chain and you can keep riding, but sometimes you'll need to stop and yank it out by hand. More than once, I've seen chain jammed so bad that the crankarm had to be removed.

Rear shifts are much less problematic. Modern derailleurs with ramped cassette cogs, which help lift the chain move, will shift even under the most extreme pedaling pressure. So go ahead and wear out that right-hand shifter. Move progressively through the gears, higher or lower, every time you sense the need. As with front shifts, anticipation is the key to maximizing momentum. Strive to keep your pedaling cadence in the efficient range between a gear that spins out and one that bogs down. When you develop your timing and shift exactly when you need to, your legs will barely feel the resistance change.

Tricky Surfaces

Rides aren't always on firm, dry trails with good traction. Let's look at several other surface conditions and how to maintain momentum on them. A primary skill for each is to use more body lean and less bike lean to get safely through turns. An upright bike reduces the risk of the tires breaking traction and sliding out. By leaning your body, you also reduce the need to steer with the handlebar. There's less chance of the front wheel plowing or slipping away.

Mud. Mud is one of the most challenging riding conditions, especially when slippery rocks and roots are also involved. It's like riding on ice but with even more painful things to fall on. To become a master of mud, you must keep your weight changes subtle and have the self-discipline to stay off the brakes.

Always try to hit wet roots at a 90-degree angle to prevent your wheels from sliding sideways. On wet rocks, try for the center or most horizontal surface, rather than a sloped side that will let your wheel slip out. Use just enough body motion both side to side and front to back to keep your weight centered between the wheels. The idea is to keep the bike as perpendicular as possible to the slippery thing you're riding over. The same is true when going around a muddy off-camber turn.

No matter how hard you try, though, there will be times when you start to slide. Then it's a matter of how quickly you can rebalance to prevent falling. Even when sliding down a slippery root, it's possible to save yourself with a swift but smooth body angulation. The best way to develop the right instincts and reaction speed is to get out there and get muddy.

Always think: Ride light. Be balanced, centered, and gentle. Riding in mud is like driving a car on an icy road. You need to be very subtle with all

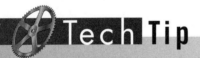

Tech Tip

During a muddy ride or race, shifting can go haywire as wet, gooey stuff coats your chain, derailleurs, and cassette. Suddenly, you can't shift into the gear you need, or the chain starts jumping or jamming. You can kiss your momentum bye-bye.

Unless, that is, you've equipped your bike with a crud claw. This is a simple, inexpensive little gizmo made by several different companies. It mounts easily on the rear axle. Its narrow fingers extend between the cassette cogs to comb out mud on each wheel revolution. It works great. I never race in the mud without one.

Derailleur covers are helpful, too. These are made of a pliable rubbery material. They slip on easily and let the derailleurs function normally while protecting them from much of the muck that the wheels throw their way. The front derailleur is especially vulnerable, so covering it is a good idea.

of your actions, especially braking, descending, turning, and accelerating. Be gradual with steering inputs. Don't exaggerate anything. Once a wheel breaks loose, the bike can get away from you really fast.

When climbing a muddy trail, stay seated so you can keep your pedal pressure as even as possible. Concentrate on pedaling in circles to smooth out your power pulses. If you don't, you'll lose rear-wheel traction. It may help to use a slightly higher gear, which makes it easier to apply pressure in all directions of your stroke. Conversely, a lower gear is more likely to cause a choppy, uneven stroke that breaks the rear wheel's grip. It's important to fight for traction and momentum on a muddy climb because once they're gone, it's real hard to get moving again. You may have to push the bike all the way to the top.

Muddy descents are challenging for several reasons. First, it might be so gooey that, even with gravity's help, you have to pedal pretty hard to keep your speed. You get no rest after the tough climb. But you can quickly get out of control if you start rolling too fast before realizing that the next bend is off-camber and the mud on your rims has increased the distance it takes to slow down. In this scenario, it helps to know the trail and whether there are steep sections or turns with rocks or roots. If so, start slower from the top. If you're riding in unfamiliar terrain, expect the worst because you'll probably get it.

If you think it's tough so far, there's one other problem that mud creates: lousy or nonexistent shifting. As mud coats the drivetrain, your hand force may be able to make shifts in one direction, but the derailleurs' return springs may get too loaded to shift the opposite way. The usual result is loss of the small chainring and the smaller cogs. Or, when you're on the smaller cogs, the chain skips because the rear derailleur is too fouled to provide enough tension. All you can do is use the middle or large chainring and hope for sufficient gears with the cogs that are available. This is a time to resort to the crossover gear (big ring/big cog). It'll probably be one of those that still work.

Sand. In sand, stay seated with your weight on the rear of the saddle. The objective is to keep your pedal strokes smooth and your front wheel light so it won't plow in. Let the handlebar float a bit by keeping your arms and hands relaxed, but don't let the front wheel wander off course. Turning inputs must be gentle. As in mud, it's better to steer by leaning your body rather than by turning the bar. Once the front wheel is turned past a certain angle, it will tend to catch and dig a furrow, immediately killing your momentum.

Ride into deep sandy sections with extra speed and a higher gear so your momentum will help carry you through. In longer sections, as your speed slows, shift down one gear at a time. The timing can be tricky. Too low a gear will cause you to bounce as you pedal and sink deeper, but you'll also bog down if you shift too late and your cadence drops.

When riding a sandy downhill, keep your weight back farther than if you were on a harder surface. It helps to pretend that the grade is steeper than it actually is. This approach will keep the front wheel very light so it's less likely to plow in. If you need to brake, go easy because you'll slow down much quicker than when on firmer ground. Any braking on sand will jeopardize your momentum.

Gravel. Gravel comes in all sizes and degrees of looseness. It can feel like you're riding on marbles or something as slippery as ice. If the gravel is loose on top of soft ground, treat it like sand. Keep your pedal strokes smooth and your cadence up, helping your tires float. Gravel on top of a hard surface can make turning treacherous. Lean your body rather than the bike, and keep steering inputs to a minimum. When in doubt, slow down. Should you slide out and crash in gravel, you'll be picking those little rocks out of your skin for days.

Snow. Snow inhibits your wheels the same as mud or sand does, so the same bike-handling techniques apply. Perhaps the biggest problem in snow is finding traction on climbs. It takes finesse to apply enough power for forward progress but not so much that the rear tire breaks traction. Sometimes, it's not entirely possible. Each pedal stroke gives you partial grip and partial slip. Move your weight farther back for more rear-tire bite and less front-tire plowing.

I like to ride on snow because it's a great way to sharpen several bike-handling skills. It improves cornering and the ability to maintain momentum. It's fun to see how far you can get up a snowy road that has tire or snowmobile tracks. You need to pedal with consistent pressure because surging will make your rear tire lose traction. You also need to maintain your line on the packed track or you'll sink into the soft snow. This is an excellent way to improve balance. Two other things I like: You're moving slow on snowy roads, so it's pretty easy to stay warm; and if you fall, you have something cushy to land on—a rare treat in this sport. It sure beats sitting on an indoor trainer all winter, too.

Ice. On ice, all bets are off. Your wheels slip away so fast that there's no time to put a foot down. You're likely to land heavily on your hip or shoulder, and that hurts. I've done it a few times on winter rides in Durango, Colorado.

So when you're cruising along and suddenly see a patch of ice, reduce speed and get a foot out. This is mandatory in a turn. Hold your inside foot to the side so you can catch yourself if the wheels suddenly slide away.

If you ride a lot on icy surfaces, equip your wheels with studded tires or chains. They work amazingly well. With chains, you can corner on ice almost as securely as you can on dirt. Northern riders can have a blast on frozen lakes.

Water. Stream crossings produce some of the best race stories. Take the watery World Cup in Plymouth, England, for instance. It's notorious for the amount of time that riders spend in its streams. The streams are always high because the race is held in late spring.

One year, David Baker and I were out in front with one-half lap to go. I was right on him. We were all set for a battle to the finish. Fatigue was coming on, though, and maybe my reflexes weren't as sharp as they should have been when I entered a long stream crossing. The water was more than 2 feet deep. I hit something with my front wheel that stopped my momentum dead. I didn't get a foot out in time and fell over, completely submerged. The crowd got a kick out of it because there I was, underwater but still on my bike. By the time I pulled myself out, David was gone. There was no way I could catch him now that I was 10 pounds heavier and freezing.

Riding into water leads to all kinds of problems that can drown your momentum. One obvious prerequisite is to judge how deep a stream is so you don't get in over your head (sometimes literally). A good example occurs on race courses like Big Bear in California. It has a stream crossing that everyone can ride on the first lap. No problem. But by the last lap, after hundreds of wheels have rolled through, there's a deep hole. Suddenly, front wheels disappear and guys go over their handlebars. It wastes a lot of time and energy to pull the bike out, remount, and get moving again.

What's the solution? In a race, watch the rider ahead of you. If he's having trouble in the stream, consider dismounting and carrying your bike across. This is quicker than waiting till you come to a stop in the water and have to climb off. Another tactic is to ride a wider line so you miss the abyss. Going off course can be risky, though, if the water is muddy and you can't see the bottom.

As you enter the water, be ready for a sudden deceleration. This braking effect throws your weight forward. To counteract it, extend your arms to push your body back. In a situation where you ride down into a stream, treat the downhill as if it's steeper than it actually is so you won't underestimate the forward weight shift.

The worst water-related momentum robber is a flat tire. A rider blasts into a shallow stream crossing, trying to keep up his speed, then hits sharp rocks on the bottom. It happens all the time. It's a common sight in races to see a guy fixing a flat on the far side of a stream. There's no way to eliminate this risk when you're trying to be competitive and you can't see rocks through the splashing of other racers. On recreational rides, simply reduce your speed, especially when riding into murky water.

Some streams present an additional problem. You churn through the water and are about to exit, only to face a steep bank. If your momentum isn't enough to carry you over, you'd better be in a gear that you can pedal. The problem is that riders forget to shift down. They stay in the same relatively high gear that they used to enter the water. They lose speed as they cross, then they can't get the gear turning again to climb out.

It's possible to shift gears in the stream, but usually you're too distracted by things like submerged riders. You need to anticipate the exit gear and shift into it before you get into this mess.

12 Unweighting

The Key to Hops, Jumps, and Other Uplifting Moves

The World Cup race in Heerlen, Holland, was just minutes from ending. We were on a flat, fast trail, twisting through the woods. Three riders had escaped. I was in the chase with four other guys, and I was cooked. My goal was to cling to their draft and hope for the best.

The trail seemed to close in. The curves and shadows made it hard to see and maneuver. Dutch rider Tommy Post was right in front of me. Suddenly, his handlebar hooked a stout little tree. He went down instantly, his bike bouncing off the trail. I knew I was going to plow into him. Instinctively, I unweighted just as I made contact. It happened so fast that he was still rolling. I couldn't get much air, but my front wheel was light enough to bounce over him rather than stick in and pivot me over my handlebar. My rear wheel hit him harder, but I kept control—and didn't lose the group.

After the race, Tommy had my tire marks etched into his thighs. We laughed about it. (I think I laughed a little harder than he did, but he's a tough guy.) The fact that I was able to do the right thing without even thinking saved both of us from plenty of damage. The lesson is that no matter what (or who) you find on the trail, unweighting is likely to be the key to the right move.

Unweighting is a technical-sounding term that's not heard a lot in recreational mountain biking. In racing, though, we use it all the time. Unweighting is at the heart of many of the sport's more advanced moves, including wheelies, bunny hops, and jumps. Have you seen guys ride up and over big logs or tall ledges? Fly their bikes above dangerous rocks? Catch big air to hurdle ditches? If so, then you've seen unweighting in action.

The term means just what it says. Normally, your weight on the bike is a constant. If you weigh 150 pounds, all 150 pounds are borne by the wheels. However, you can lighten this load (unweight) for brief but crucial moments by combining shifts in body position with lifting or pulling with your arms and legs.

The possibilities are amazing. Look at the jumps that kids can do on their BMX bikes even without their feet attached to the pedals by cleats or toe straps. Watch what happens when stuntmen like Hans Rey ride up to a picnic table or junked car. They ride over it just about as easily as the rest of us handle a tall curb. Such is the power of unweighting.

Three major moves made possible by unweighting are wheelies, bunny hops, and jumps. Wheelies are the easiest to execute and bunny hops are the most difficult. Realize, though, that sometimes unweighting is a subtle move that is not intended to get you off the ground. All you need to do is lighten your wheels so they don't strike too hard on something (just ask Tommy Post). The basic unweight maneuver lets you load and unload to skim the bike over small obstacles. This is useful on a trail with short rough sections that may cause pinch flats. Instead of plowing through and absorbing all the jolts or using extra energy to jump the bike, you can unweight to let the wheels bounce along lightly and keep you in control.

A word of caution, though: The following techniques can result in falls and injuries. One of my pals at *Bicycling* magazine went over backward while practicing wheelies in the parking lot before a ride. Even though he's an expert bike handler, he lost it. The result was a back injury that plagued him for months. Always wear your helmet and practice initially on a soft, forgiving surface like a grassy field.

Wheelies

When you hear "wheelie," you probably think of showing off—pulling up the front of the bike and pedaling along on the rear wheel. This isn't the kind of wheelie that's used in trail riding, though it is a good advanced drill for improving balance. Two other types of wheelies are much more essential. They're the key to getting up and over logs, ledges, or similar obstacles.

The first is what I call the power-stroke wheelie. Normally, you use this

Deep in your heart, you'd probably like to be able to ride an extended wheelie. I'll tell you how because if you learn, it'll increase your mastery of the bike, which is always a good thing. And, yeah, it'll impress the heck out of your riding buddies, too.

First, you need to respect the fact that when you're balancing on the rear wheel, you're on the brink of tipping over backward. Practice on a soft, forgiving surface and wear your helmet. If you start tilting too far back, react quickly by tapping your rear brake, lightening pedal pressure, or leaning forward. If these remedies don't work, don't hang on—step off the rear of the bike. Keep your feet loose on the pedals (not clipped in) so you can get them down immediately.

Begin with a power stroke. Push down hard on one pedal, shift your weight backward, pull back on the handlebar, and use the saddle as a lever to raise the front of the bike. This lofts the front wheel. Be in a gear that's high enough to let you keep constant pressure on the pedals. If you build up too much speed, you'll spin out, but you can shift to a bigger gear with your front wheel still in the air. You're jammin' now.

Your goal is to find and maintain the balance point. In this way, an extended wheelie is kind of like a trackstand. It helps to cross up your front wheel (like in a jump) by turning the handlebar a bit one way or the other while airborne, stick out a knee, twist your shoulders—anything goes if it prolongs your rear-wheel equilibrium. When the front wheel comes back down, make sure it's pointed straight ahead.

Personally, I can't ride an extended wheelie worth beans. It's just not a skill I developed, and it isn't a prerequisite for being a good bike handler. But I do sometimes practice because it helps my balance and technical riding. It makes it easier to relax and feel comfortable when the front wheel is in the air, like during hops and jumps.

when approaching at a relatively slow speed. The technique is to push down hard on one pedal, shift your weight backward, pull back on the handlebar, and use the saddle as a sort of lever to raise the front of the bike. It may sound kind of difficult, but it becomes second nature with practice. What you need to work on is the tendency to overdo the bar pull while giving insufficient emphasis to the other elements. That's the mistake that most riders make.

The power-stroke wheelie is actually a leverage move that requires very little arm action. It's more a matter of holding on to the bar and leaning back as you apply the power stroke. The rearward lean, rather than arm action by itself, is what pulls up the front of the bike. Remember, the pull and

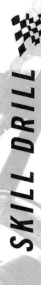

No discussion of wheelies is complete without including the nose wheelie— balancing on the front wheel alone. I'll describe it because I want you to know every important technique, but as you can imagine, it's very risky. You can easily tip forward onto your head, or the front wheel can slide out if you grab too much front brake in an area with loose traction.

You're going to get into this position on the trail now and then, so you should become familiar with it in controlled conditions and develop the right reactions. Unintentional nose wheelies can happen when you brake too hard or bump into something at slow speed. The risk is greater on downhills, when your weight is naturally forward.

Practice on soft stuff with your helmet on. Roll straight ahead at slow speed, stand, extend your arms to move your weight back, then lock the front brake. As the rear of the bike comes up, let the saddle pass between your legs. (You can lower it for this drill.) Now you're stopped dead, balanced on the front wheel.

Try to remain balanced for a couple of seconds (it'll seem a lot longer). Start by lifting the rear wheel a couple of inches, then build on this as you become more comfortable perched on the front wheel. When a nose wheelie happens inadvertently, this practice will help you calmly deal with it by shifting your weight farther back and reducing your grip on the front-brake lever.

You can let the rear wheel drop straight back to the ground so you can put a foot down to prevent a fall. Or you can pivot the rear of the bike to one side, angling it on a new course so you can ride away. That's a very cool move.

---

sharp downstroke must be simultaneous. Make sure you're in a gear that's low enough to let you make the stroke quickly and get some pop. As the front wheel clears the object, shift your weight forward. Resume pedaling after the rear wheel makes contact, then return to your normal centered position. It's important to practice power-stroke wheelies with each foot so you'll have the option on a tricky trail.

Next is the wheelie hop. Use this when your approach speed is faster. In this situation, you don't need to use a power stroke to start the wheelie. Just loft the front wheel with a rearward pull, land it on top of the obstacle, then surge your body weight forward so you bring up the rear wheel. As the front wheel rolls off, the rear wheel lands on top, then easily follows.

If you have trouble with these wheelies, it's probably because you force them. Think "leverage" instead of "power." Rather than yanking back on the handlebar to get the front wheel up, lean backward so the bike pivots around the crankset. These wheelies become easy when you lift the bike with a weight shift instead of with your arm strength. You'll know you're using the right technique when it seems almost effortless.

Bunny Hops

The bunny hop is an exaggerated unweight combined with sucking the bike up into your body for maximum height and distance. It's especially useful for totally clearing objects such as logs, rocks, curbs, or small animals when riding with some speed. When you don't want your wheels to touch an obstacle, or when you want to get your bike up onto something high, you bunny hop. This move also avoids the chainring damage that can occur when using a wheelie to get over a large rock or ledge.

Most mere mortals, myself included, need some forward momentum to initiate a bunny hop. But some trials riders have developed the ability to jump 5 feet or more straight up from a trackstand. You don't need such skill

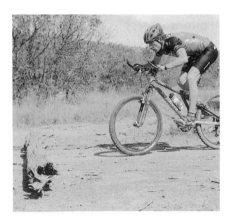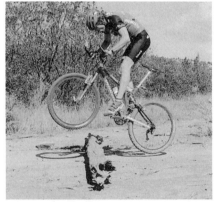

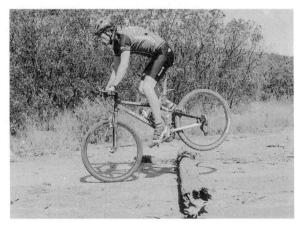

To bunny hop over an obstacle, approach in the attack position with enough momentum to get you across. Stop pedaling, and press into the bike to load it like a spring (top left). Unweight to lift off, pulling up the front wheel with your arms (top right). Push the front wheel forward and suck up your legs to lift the rear wheel over (bottom).

87

or altitude for cross-country riding, but the ability to bunny hop 1 or 2 feet should be within everyone's ability.

In unweighting for bunny hopping, your body acts like a spring. You load by pressing down on the handlebar and pedals, then pop upward. But there are additional motions in a bunny hop that many riders have trouble understanding. I'll clue you in, then you have to go practice by hopping over soft things (like a cardboard box or a bag of leaves) that won't cause a problem if you goof.

Begin with your weight centered and your crankarms horizontal, and with a bit of speed. Make a quick crouch to load the bike, pressing down on the handlebar and pedals to compress the "springs" in your arms and legs. Lift the front wheel first, not both wheels together (a common mistake). As the front wheel comes up, push the bar away and roll your wrists downward as you suck your legs up toward your body. This action brings up the rear wheel. Pull in your legs as tight as you can to gain maximum height.

If you stand back and watch a good bunny hopper, you'll see a snaking motion. The front wheel comes up and then arcs forward. It's a technique based on fluid finesse, not power. When I teach bunny hopping at a camp, most riders initially make the mistake of jerking the front wheel up. They get very little air because they fail to suck the bike upward and push it forward. Think of bunny hopping as launching your body. Once the front end of the bike is in the air, bring the bike through by pushing with your arms, rolling your wrists, and pulling up with your legs.

Jumps

You can ride over an amazing array of obstacles on a mountain bike. And I do mean *over*. Jumping lets you fly past many things that you'd rather not have your wheels touch. This is a relatively high-speed technique. And like the other unweighting moves, it relies on finesse and timing rather than on brute strength.

Jumping is exhilarating and a valuable part of any rider's arsenal, but remember to do it with caution. There can be a serious price to pay if you do a lot of jumping, because sooner or later you're going to throw yourself onto the ground. This brings to mind the NORBA Nationals course in Traverse City, Michigan, with its infamous water jump. This thing is a real crowd pleaser. It bags a few collarbones and an occasional femur every year. The pool is about 10 feet long with a ramp at one end and a sharp lip at the other. You can swallow your pride and ride around it, or you can pedal as hard as you can in your highest gear and jump it. Most guys who go for it actually do clear the water, but some of them crash anyway because they land off-balance. Cross-country riders aren't used to being in the air for that long, so they sometimes wind up doing what we call a dead sailor. While in the air, they get rigid, and they start tilting to the side. I know quite a few guys who've crashed for this reason.

To maintain orientation during a jump, I like to "cross up" my front wheel by turning the handlebar a bit one way or the other while airborne. You'll see BMXers, motocross racers, and other hotshots do it. It's not just for show. If you cross up the front wheel and then straighten it for the landing, you have something to do up there. You have a reference that helps you maintain your trajectory. You're not just a stiff missile. Try this technique, and you'll find it easier to stay centered for your landings. Just be sure to have the front wheel pointed straight again before you touch down.

The basic skill in becoming airborne is—you guessed it—unweighting the bike. You also need speed to create momentum and preserve the wheels' gyroscopic effect that helps your control. Launch from the attack position, in which you are off the saddle, crouched, with your weight centered and crankarms horizontal (see chapter 2 for more information). Think of your legs as springs. Press down to load them, then pounce. Suck the bike into your body if you want to maximize height and distance.

Timing your launch depends on your speed, so it's a matter of practice. The faster you go, the sooner you need to start preparing to unweight. Begin by jumping low, safe obstacles with a gradual launching ramp. Small bumps are ideal. You'll find that you can't unweight for a jump in a turn, because you need the traction. You simply have to slow down and use other techniques to get past obstacles.

Words of Wisdom

As a cross-country rider, I've spent lots of time trying to keep my wheels on the ground. But for some reason, since I turned 40, I've been enjoying jumps more and more. I've also been influenced by Greg Herbold, a good friend and former world downhill champion who has incredible bike-handling ability, especially when he's going really fast and getting air. Here are some of his jumping secrets.

"Before you start working on your technique, it's very important to find a jump with a nice smooth approach, a gradual and gentle lip, and a smooth landing and runout area. Trying to practice jumps in a place not well-designed for jumps will only lead to hospital visits.

"The most important thing in the approach is to have a smooth line. You don't want to be making any late adjustments. Be sure you have a good view of the place from which you're going to launch. Then, the key to the takeoff is to be centered on your bike, fore and aft and side to side. Bend your elbows. Bend your knees slightly. Be in position to react in any way necessary when your bike hits that bump.

"The third thing is what you do in the air. Mountain bikers have a tendency to be cast-iron statues. Instead, you want to be loose, flexible, and looking where you're going. Turning or crossing up your front wheel helps orient you, but you have to get it straight again before you land.

"Landing takes a little practice. Usually, the smoothest landings are rear wheel first or at least both wheels together. The main thing you want to avoid is a front-wheel landing, which can cause an endo."

Despite the fact that jumping is second nature to Greg, it's not necessarily the safest, fastest, or easiest way for most of us to stay in control on rough terrain. Often, it's better to suck up the big bumps to avoid becoming airborne and changing trajectory. Assume the attack position and use your arms and legs to force the bike along the contour of the terrain, keeping your torso fairly quiet. Sharply pull up and push down the front wheel to maintain contact and control. Be ready with your arsenal of wheelies and bunny hops. After you've mastered these moves, you'll be able to ride over almost anything.

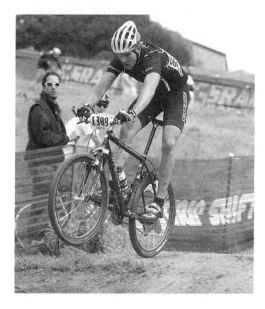

When landing from a jump, touch down on the rear wheel first or both wheels together. Keep your weight back and bend your knees and elbows to absorb the impact.

13 Steep Climbs

Techniques for Traction When the Trail Gets Vertical

At the 1990 world championship in Durango, Colorado, Thomas Frischknecht and I were locked in a dogfight. For three laps we battled, leaving the field far behind. One of us would become mountain biking's first-ever gold medalist. The other would become a footnote. On this day, the difficulty of the course would be the deciding factor.

At the start of the fourth and final lap was a pitch of rocky, loose trail that went straight up the face of a ski run. Steep? Vertical, or so it seemed after two hours of racing at 9,500 feet. My Swiss rival had been dismounting and running this climb while I stayed on my bike. On previous laps, I'd opened a little gap, so I knew this would be my chance. I attacked when Thomas got off again. He never caught me. My dream came true—I won the sport's biggest race, and it happened in my hometown.

To ride that steep trail, I had to use five climbing techniques. There's no reason why you can't make them part of your arsenal, too.

Pedal in circles. If you only hammer downward on the pedals, this jerky power transmission will break your rear-tire traction and rob momentum. If this had happened to me in the world championship, I would have had to get off and run with Thomas. As a star cyclocross racer, he would have gained the advantage—and probably the gold medal, too.

To develop a smooth stroke that maintains traction, you need to master

91

the four phases of pedaling, which are covered in chapter 3. Two phases are worth reemphasizing here because they're so essential to strong climbing. First, when your foot approaches the bottom of the stroke, start dragging it backward like you're scraping mud from your shoe. Keep the sole parallel to the ground. Then, instead of merely pulling up, drive your knee toward the handlebar. This helps you come across the top of the pedal circle and smoothly begin the next downstroke.

A good drill on a mild incline is to unclip a foot and hold it to the side so you can pedal with one leg and then the other. This teaches you the feeling of pedaling through the top and bottom.

Shift your weight. Climbing while seated requires a smooth pedal stroke plus a front-to-rear balancing act. Bend at the waist, lowering your chest toward the handlebar to weight the front wheel and prevent it from getting light and wandering or popping up. For more traction in back, raise your chest. Combine this down-and-up movement with sliding fore and aft

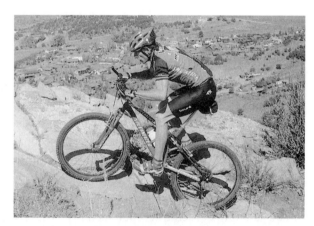

Whether you're tackling a steep climb in the saddle (top) or standing (bottom), two rules apply. First, lean low and pull the handlebar with your elbows down to prevent the front wheel from popping up. Second, keep your butt back so there's enough weight over the rear wheel to maintain traction.

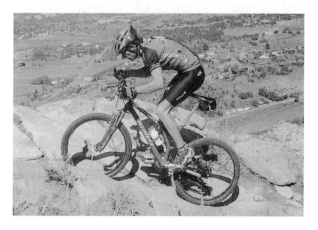

on the saddle. The goal is an ideal balance between rear-wheel power traction and front-wheel steering traction. This is critical for steep climbing, because at slow speed you don't have the gyroscopic effect of the wheels to help hold the bike upright. By practicing very slow riding, you can improve your sense of balance. Then you can turn your concentration to weight shifts for traction and steering.

Stand and deliver. I rise from the saddle when I need to generate more climbing power. This allows me to incorporate more back and shoulder muscles to increase rear-wheel traction. Start with a smooth transition from your sitting position. Don't stand straight up as you do on a road bike. Stay bent at the waist with your butt just in front of and above the nose of the saddle. Picture your pelvis as a fulcrum, with your hands and handlebar at one end and the rear tire at the other. By pulling back (not up) on the bar, you can leverage the rear tire into the dirt. Bar-ends increase this leverage effect, so I recommend installing a pair if you haven't already.

Because standing uses more energy, do it sparingly to get through the crux of a climb or for a sudden burst of speed. Otherwise, it's more efficient to stay seated.

Pick a line. Scan the trail for the best traction. In a race, often the best line will change if there's a lot of traffic, so it doesn't always work to use the same line every lap. You may find the best traction on the edge of the trail, not quite in the grass but beside the section where other riders have loosened the dirt.

Avoiding obstacles such as large rocks and ruts is easier the farther you plan ahead. This lets you change direction gradually without sacrificing climbing traction. Reading the terrain will help you shift to the proper gear ahead of time so you're not trying to find traction, steer around rocks, and grab an easier gear all at once.

Select the right gear. Different riders are comfortable with different pedaling cadences. One common mistake is to choose a gear that's too high. This can cause you to bog down, lose momentum, and put a foot down on the steep technical sections. Conversely, many riders shift to lower gears too soon on a climb, losing momentum on the transition from gradual to steep. Of course, you should shift to the smallest chainring just before you begin to lose momentum and heavy pedal pressure increases the risk of chainsuck. But if you shift too early, you'll be bouncing at the base of the climb with a cadence that's too high. You won't be able to put enough pressure on the pedals for a smooth stroke—goodbye traction.

Ned's KNOWLEDGE

Lots of steep climbs are also high climbs. I live in Durango, Colorado, at 6,500 feet above sea level but have often competed on alpine courses at 9,000 feet or higher. Believe me, the effect on performance is significant.

Let's look at what you should expect when you find yourself riding at an altitude that is thousands of feet higher than where you live. Experts say the effects start to become very noticeable at about 6,500 feet.

First, let's clear up a common misconception. The reason it's harder to breathe at high altitude isn't because there's less oxygen. The air's oxygen concentration is about 21 percent whether you're on the beach in Miami or on top of Mount Everest. What is drastically different is the amount of atmospheric pressure, which is what forces oxygen into your lungs. The higher you go, the lower the pressure. Your lungs and heart must work harder to meet your body's oxygen demands.

You'll notice this when doing something as simple as walking upstairs at the high-altitude mountain bike meccas. Now go for a ride. You'll breathe harder, fatigue faster, and perform worse—at least during the three or four weeks that it takes to become acclimated. The trouble is, vacations or trips to races rarely last long enough for you to adjust.

Some riders suffer more than others. I'm convinced that it's often a matter of attitude rather than altitude. Take my old pal and fellow racer Steve Tilford, for instance. This guy is as hard as nails. The tougher the race, the more he loves it—except when it's at altitude. Then he whines like a three-year-old at the doctor's office. He says high-altitude races are unfair. He's sure he won't do well, so he usually doesn't. On the other side is pro racer Tinker Juarez, who rides great in high altitude despite being from Los Angeles.

For riders like Steve and Tinker, it's mostly mental. After all, nearly everyone in the race has to deal with the same problem. Very few riders actually live and train year-round at 9,000 feet. You can cope with the challenges more successfully (and develop a more positive attitude) by following the rules I use.

Remain calm. You'll be panting so hard so often that you'll fear you're in deep trouble. Look around. Everyone else is sucking wind, too. Here's a trick: Exhale forcefully and inhale passively to maintain effective breathing. This technique is favored by Olympic road champion Alexi Grewal, who hails from the high mountains of Aspen, Colorado.

Eat well. You may not have a great appetite, but keep eating on the bike and between rides. Your body works harder at altitude and needs more calories.

Drink lots of water. You're at risk of dehydration because your respiration rate is up and most high-altitude locations are also very dry. You'll feel even greater fatigue if you don't replace all of the fluid you're losing.

Cut down on alcohol and caffeine. These are diuretics, so they make it harder to stay hydrated. Some riders, myself included, experience more frequent urination at altitude even without ingesting these substances.

Reduce riding intensity. If you immediately try to ride at 9,000 feet like you do at sea level, you'll bury yourself and it will take days to recover. This may be worth it for a one-day race, but it will sure ruin a vacation. Going hard too soon also puts you at risk of altitude sickness, marked by headache, nausea, and major malaise. You may have to go to a lower altitude to recover.

Race on the first day or after the fourth day. Some riders have success by showing up and competing almost before their bodies realize what's happening. On the flip side, several days of training at altitude will probably make you tired. By the fifth day, you should be acclimated enough to feel normal again. True adaptation takes at least three weeks, according to the experts.

Beware of a raspy cough. In high, dry conditions you can develop pulmonary edema, or fluid in the lungs. This can be dangerous, so consider going to a lower altitude and seeing a doctor if this develops.

Rest more. I'm talking about time in bed as well as time between steep climbs or other hard efforts. Unless you're racing, avoid going anaerobic. Pace yourself and allow extra time for recovery.

Finally, you're probably wondering if you will ride better when you get back home. It's not likely after only a week or two at altitude. In fact, you may have less fitness because you weren't able to ride as hard or as long. That's the reason for a technique that's being used by some elite cyclists and runners. They train at lower altitude so they can push their bodies harder, then they go up the mountain to sleep and obtain the three main physiological adaptations to high altitude: an increase in oxygen-carrying red blood cells, larger lungs to help more oxygen enter the bloodstream, and a bigger heart and larger blood vessels to transport the oxygen to muscles.

All of these things help cycling performance, but they take months or years to fully develop. Rather than expect a boost from your occasional trip to the mountains, just do what you can to neutralize the potential stresses. Enjoy the challenges—and the views.

Lessons for Long Climbs

Now, let's see how to handle a climb that's not only fairly steep but that also goes on and on. We have plenty of these on the NORBA race circuit. Long climbs yield plenty of lessons, so I always try to learn from my mistakes. For instance, consider what happened at a Grundig World Cup race in Vail, Colorado. I went into it with good fitness and lots of (too much) confidence. It should have been one of my best performances, but instead it was one of the worst because I ignored much of what I'd learned through the years.

You have to respect long hard climbs, especially at high altitude. I'd previously won the World Cup final on the same course and was determined to win there again. But unlike earlier, when I started steady and picked my way through the field, this time I charged from the gun to fight with the early leaders. Fifteen minutes into the race, I was telling myself, "Back off. You're breathing too hard and putting too much pressure on your legs in the steep sections." I was intoxicated by the crowd's cheers, battling with the leaders, and putting time on the rest of the field. I was staying close to the front but at too high of a price.

After 90 minutes, I was about to blow. I knew it was curtains when I began planning alternative careers and thinking about how nice it would be if I weren't sponsored so I could just ride back to my car and make a sandwich. I suffered like a dog while a good chunk of the field paraded by. I eventually finished 25th. It would have been worse, except half the field blew up with me.

So what lessons should I have remembered before the start gun went off and rendered me a moron? And what lessons can you learn, even if you don't race? Here are the most important.

Go out easy. Long climbs don't require high-speed starts (especially on a hot day at 8,500 feet). Pacing is all-important, even on weekend jaunts. Chances are very good that your fast-starting pals will come back to you later. In a race, count on seeing the jackrabbits again in the second half. Big time gaps are quickly erased when riders have to resort to crawling on their hands and knees.

Use experience to dictate a realistic pace. Factor in the length and steepness of the climbs, plus heat, humidity, and altitude. If it's a race and you can preride the course, try to estimate your finishing time, then determine a pace based on your level of fitness.

Relax and establish a rhythm. Don't contract muscles that aren't being used to move you forward. Many riders have a tendency to tighten their jaws and necks when they climb, and this often extends to their chests. It's critical that your chest be relaxed so it can expand easily. You pull back on the handlebar in rhythm with your pedaling downstroke on each side. This requires a firm hold on the bar, but not a death grip. The trick is to pull on the bar without using every muscle in your upper body. Practice in training by using your bar for leverage while contracting as few muscles in your arms and shoulders as necessary. I like to give a forceful exhale every couple of minutes as a cue to relax. And remember to stay seated whenever possible. This uses less energy because you don't have to support your body weight.

Heed your body's warning signs. When you know you're running low on energy, start to ride defensively, using lower gears and taking in more calories and fluids. I try to drink a 20-ounce bottle every half-hour, whether I'm thirsty or not. If you do blow, slow down, recover, and parcel what's left of your energy to the finish.

14 Rapid Descents

Seven Ways to Boost Downhill Skill

One fascinating thing about great downhill racers is that they don't look fast. They're fluid. They're relaxed. They simply do everything right and eliminate the excesses. They corner without locking their brakes and scrubbing off more speed than they need to. They suck up bumps instead of being pitched into the air by them. In fact, they stay on the ground as much as possible. You may assume it's faster to fly the bike, but remember, if you're airborne, you can't turn or do anything else until you come back down.

What you don't see from the best descenders is a lot of slipping and sliding around. Those things only make you seem like you're fast. Sometimes, you can't avoid getting launched by a bump, but skilled downhillers know how to limit even this. They "prejump" the bump by unweighting before they reach its front lip, essentially making a small jump over the lip to avoid being launched into the air by it. This carries them to a landing just on the other side after minimal air time.

Why is this important? Because a turn or rough section might be coming right up. If they arrive in the air, they won't have time to choose the best line, and they could even pinch flat or break a wheel by coming down on rocks.

Suspension Is Key

Now you can understand why lots of suspension is beneficial on downhill bikes. Current models come with as much as 5 to 8 inches of front- and rear-suspension travel. This helps keep the tires on the ground for better traction, braking, and turning, while reducing pinch flats and rider fatigue. Suspension also reduces the risk of breaking a frame, a common problem in the days of rigid bikes and even on hardtails (bikes with front but no rear suspension). Of course, now the concern has switched to the durability of the suspension. I see more failures in shock systems than in any other parts of bikes (except inner tubes).

If you're still riding a hardtail, it's safe to say that nothing can improve your downhilling as much as going to a dual-suspension bike, or dualie. It's a huge help. A dualie enables you to increase speed and safety simultaneously because your tires stay on the ground much more. Imagine what happens in a rough, rutty, off-camber turn. If the dual suspension is set up properly, the tires follow the contour of the ground and stay on the desired line. If not, they buck and bounce into the air. When they come down, they're farther toward the outside of the turn, thanks to centrifugal force. This jeopardizes control and costs time.

I encourage you to experiment with your bike's suspension. There are many different systems, so it's up to you to become thoroughly familiar with your specific equipment. Read the owner's manual and try different adjustments. Consider your riding style, terrain, and ability, not just your weight. In this way, suspension tuning is just like a riding skill. You need to get the information, then apply it to your specific situation. As rides go by, service your shocks and readjust them as necessary for optimum performance. Suspension response changes with hard use.

In general, you want the best trade-off between your shocks' abilities to absorb small bumps and big jumps. You want to set your shocks' rebound damping to be light enough for your wheels to react quickly to the ground's contours. But if it's too light, it won't slow the return spring, making it feel like you're riding a pogo stick. If you're a cross-country racer, you may want to sacrifice some of the suspension's suppleness in order to make it more efficient (that is, less active). Or you may choose to give up a little efficiency on climbs by making the suspension supple enough to help you rip the descents. Keep tweaking and evaluating the results. Don't just accept the settings that came with your bike. (For a full discussion of suspension, see chapter 10.)

Look Before You Leap

Vision is key to descending. The faster you go, the faster things happen. If you're always concentrating on the trail right in front of you, it severely limits your speed—or at least how fast you can safely go. Instead, you should scan the terrain, looking up to the farthest point on your horizon for new developments. Put your brain into cataloging mode. Your thought process may go like this: "Turn coming up, . . . brake here, . . . watch that rut, . . . quick unweight, . . . twist, . . . catch that berm. . . . "

What is really remarkable is that you can do all this without actually thinking. By understanding descending techniques and then practicing them, your moves will become instinctive as your eyes supply the details. This is how you want to ride all the time, of course, but on downhills, it's even more crucial. The more you practice, the more ingrained the correct reflexes become.

I, for instance, had to get rid of the tendency to grab the front brake in turns, especially off-camber turns with loose surfaces. This tendency was a recipe for front-wheel washouts. I broke the braking habit by getting into a different habit—extending my left fingers straight ahead when in the apex of such a turn. This once-conscious remedy is now automatic.

Even the very best downhillers aren't immune to bad habits. I was fortunate that it took several years for pro racer John Tomac to get over his. When he came to mountain biking from BMX, he forced everyone to ride faster, primarily by descending faster. I absolutely had to improve my downhilling if I was going to get back on top, which is where I was before John arrived. He and I had some classic battles. I eventually won six cross-country national championships, and every one of them was against him. He beat me in two others.

Ironically, I owe more than one victory to John's mistakes on downhills. Bike handling at high speed was natural to him, but this also made him very hard on equipment. He trashed lots of bike parts because he was always getting air and landing on hard things. I can remember him complaining about a cracked frame that knocked him out of a race, but he overlooked the fact that he'd just flown 15 feet and landed in a rocky section. Or he'd run insufficient tire pressure for his speed and pinch flat on something he didn't see in time. He got so much practice fixing flats that he could change a tube and be riding again in less than two minutes.

John actually won more often when he started slowing down and riding within his vision. As his finesse increased, so did the reliability of his equipment. It's funny how that works. Before he slowed down, he spent a lot of time passing me and inadvertently teaching me how to descend faster. I got better by following him—watching his line, his cornering, his body angulation—and I started losing less time to him on downhills. When you ride with good descenders, watch them and take advantage of an excellent learning opportunity.

Take Control

The bottom line on getting to the bottom is that you're going to need almost every bike-handling skill that is discussed in this book, plus one more ingredient—relaxation. Your moves must come fluidly because things happen quickly. Practice is the best teacher. Here are seven specific things that you can do to boost your control and confidence when gravity says, "Come on down!"

1. Ride light. Envision your bike floating freely beneath you while your torso and head remain calm. To make this happen, you must avoid gripping the handlebar too hard and creating tightness that travels up your arms to your shoulders. This tension slows reaction time and increases fatigue. Instead, keep a firm grip without crushing the bar, and keep your elbows bent.

Also, stand on steep descents and use your bent knees as shock absorbers. Think of your body as making a cone of movement. If you stand, the cone (extending upward from your feet) can cover a much larger area, both laterally and vertically. But if you stay seated, movement is restricted. Experience the difference while riding on flat ground. Stand and move all around the bike. Then use this technique on downhills.

Another important benefit of standing is that it lowers your center of gravity. When you're sitting, your weight is on the saddle. When you're standing, it's on your feet. Your center of gravity moves downward, which makes a huge difference to your stability.

Riding light also helps spare your bike from damage. Let's say you're on a trail that has lots of rocks or roots. Try to equalize the weight on your wheels. Many riders tend to put more weight on the rear wheel, which is a recipe for pinch flats. The exception comes on a steep descent. Here, you must shift your weight back so the front wheel can roll over obstacles and you won't be pitched over the handlebar by front-braking forces.

If there's a good landing area, bunny hop small obstacles by compressing your knees and then unweighting to launch up and over, as described in chapter 12. Practice your timing and technique on safe objects before moving to a descent. Land gently on the rear wheel or on both wheels together. A heavy front-wheel landing on a downhill can easily pitch you over the handlebar.

2. Sink the saddle. To descend well, you need the biggest cone of movement that you can create. That's why downhill racers lower their saddles. If a saddle is in its regular cross-country–riding position, it's harder to move on the bike or shift your center of gravity. Of course, you can't pedal as efficiently with a low saddle, but for learning purposes, on steep descents I recommend moving it down several inches. (This makes it easier to bail out, too.) As you practice, you'll feel big improvements in your control and confidence. Then put the saddle back to normal height and ride the same section some more. Easier, isn't it?

3. Pick a line. When you enter a turn, centrifugal force becomes the enemy, pulling you and your tires to the outside. The first way to combat this is to "straighten" the curve by starting wide, cutting to the apex, then finishing wide. Obviously, trail conditions may not permit this every time, but the fastest line is usually the one that requires the least lean.

For precise steering control, you need a firm grip on the bar, but not a death grip. Finesse requires smooth steering inputs. Relaxed arms will help you shift your weight to put the bike onto the line you want. I see too many riders go where the bike wants to go. You must always be in charge of where the bike is going.

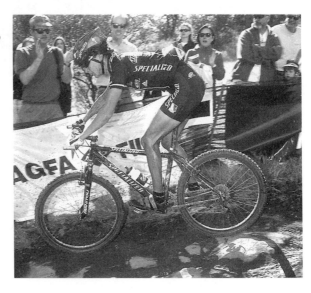

To get the most speed downhill, the best line is the smoothest one. Often, it'll be along the edge of the trail, where rocks and roots aren't exposed.

4. Brake away. It seems simplistic to say that if you want to go fast downhill, get off the brakes. But braking is more complicated than that. When you're off the brakes, not only do you roll faster but you also have greater command of the bike. This is because traction and control are reduced when the brakes are on, especially when you're turning, or riding over ruts or obstacles.

The key to avoiding the negative aspects is to stay off the brakes as much as possible, then use them in the right places. Generally, these are firm, smooth areas that you encounter when the bike is vertical. Once again, vision plays a big role. You need to spot these braking areas in time to use them—there won't be very many on most trails, and they probably won't be very large. On descents, you need the confidence to brake as hard as necessary when you find them.

Why confidence? Because a dangerous nose wheelie can easily happen. On a steep downhill, all of your braking power is at the front wheel and all of your weight moves forward. The rear wheel can get so light that it leaves the ground. This happens in downhill races all the time. It's not a problem if you have the right reactions to a nose wheelie, so review my advice in chapter 12.

Downhill racers have a straightforward strategy about braking. I think that cross-country riders would do well to copy it. It goes like this: Use the front brake to control speed; use the rear brake primarily to con-

This is a nose wheelie. It can happen during a descent when you grab too much front brake or stick an object with your front wheel. Practice nose wheelies on flat, smooth ground to learn how to push your weight way back and stay in control.

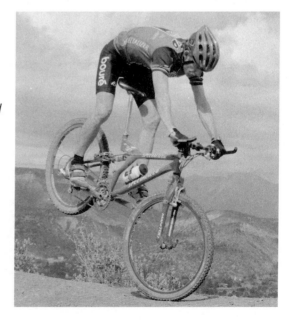

To be a better descender, you need to get comfortable with the wheel drift that is caused by centrifugal force pulling the bike off-line in a fast turn. It's also important to learn how body angulation affects turning. Once you experience the sensation, the right reactions become more instinctive.

It's important to find a good place for this training where you can practice and learn the limits of traction without much danger of a bad crash. Ideally, it will be a hillside dirt road that offers both left and right downhill turns. You want them to be pretty sharp, between 75 and 90 degrees. If necessary, create turns of the correct arc by laying down a row of stones. The road surface should be smooth, not rutted or bumpy. You need to concentrate on how your body position affects traction.

Go around and around this course. Experiment. Try turning with the crankarms horizontal, to see how unstable this feels. You need to go pretty slow because you can't lean very much. Consider this your baseline. Then try it with the outside pedal down and your weight pressing on it. Better, right? The harder you stand on the outside pedal, the more you will force the tire knobs into the dirt for a firmer grip.

Next, get your weight off the saddle. Brace the inner thigh of your outside leg against it. Angle your upper body to the outside of the turn to push the bike down into it. The result is a relatively upright body and an angled bike. Now you're really carving. You can use this technique at high speed when traction is good. If it's slippery, you'll need to compensate by reducing speed, accentuating your body angulation, and reducing the bike's lean angle.

Go through these practice turns again and again, left and right, faster and faster. If it's a left turn, push down on the handlebar with your right hand to increase front-tire traction (vice versa for a right turn). Keep your body angled to the outside.

When you reach the speed where the tires begin to drift, take your inside foot off the pedal and use your leg like an outrigger. Lean forward a bit. I ride this way more and more, because it works. It makes you less likely to crash, so your sense of security and confidence increases. You learn to let the wheels drift without panicking.

Experience the many dynamics. You can lean right or left to alter tire bite or drift. You can lean forward or backward to change the traction of the front or rear tire. For example, if you're going through a left turn and feel the front tire start to wash out, lower your chest and push down with your right hand to press the front tire harder into the dirt.

It's hard to learn these moves during a regular trail ride, when you pass through a turn just once and an aggressive mistake can be costly. This is why I'm so keen on practicing in a controlled situation. It'll make a huge improvement in your downhill turning ability.

SKILL DRILL

trol direction. Use both brakes together to take off a lot of speed in a straightaway before a turn. Regulate wheel lock-up by modulating your pull on the lever. A slight adjustment in finger pressure can mean the difference between a wheel that's skidding and one that's still turning.

The idea is to brake hard in places where you have traction, then be off the brakes on rough, loose, slippery sections. It's so much easier to get through tight turns and gnarly places when you're not braking at all. Confidence in braking ability is a major key to fast downhills.

5. Weight the outside pedal. If there's good traction in a turn or a berm is present, simply keep your upper body in line with the bike and pedal through. But in most cases, you need to coast, put your outside pedal down, press it hard, and push the bike into the turn while keeping your body angled toward the vertical. It may look to bystanders like you're sitting on the saddle, but your butt should actually be elevated slightly. All of your weight and force has to be on your outside leg to push the tires into the ground so they won't slide out. At the same time, apply downward pressure on the outside handlebar grip to add weight to the front tire. This increases its bite in the dirt.

To fly down a hill, you need to get comfortable with front- and rear-wheel drift. Wheel drift happens when centrifugal force pulls you off-line in a turn. You'll experience it often if you're descending at top speed.

6. Maintain focus. This is another good spot to remind you of a classic piece of advice: Look where you want the bike to go, not where you're afraid it may go. In Durango, Colorado, for instance, lots of trails have ravines falling away to one side and steep hills on the other. In such a situation, it's hard not to look into the chasm. But if you do, you edge that way, which makes you overcorrect and ride up the slope. You then overcorrect again and end up where you don't want to be—in the gulch. If you focus on the center of the trail, that's where you'll stay.

There are also trails that are like foot-wide islands between two ruts. If it were a painted stripe on the road, you'd have no problem staying on it. But most riders tend to look at the ruts and fall into them.

7. Stay mentally relaxed. Going fast down a tough trail can be scary. Fear is good if it makes you a little more cautious, but it also creates tenseness that can slow your reaction time. When you feel this happening, exhale forcefully to release this stress. Be conscious of gritting your teeth and tensing your neck and shoulders. When you're relaxed, you're better able to adjust quickly and fluidly to challenging situations.

15 High-Speed Turns

It's All in How You Angle Your Body

Turning may depend on more variables than any other mountain biking technique. Every turn is different and each can change within itself. Is the next turn banked, flat, or off-camber? Uphill or downhill? How wide is the arc; how tight is the track? What type of traction will the tires have?

To make it even more challenging, the same turn requires different techniques at different speeds. When you turn at low speed, the lack of gyroscopic energy in your wheels means you have to rely on balance to stay upright. On the other hand, while at high speed, you need to deal with centrifugal force. The upshot is that you need to master two distinct methods of turning: (1) turning the handlebar to steer through slow-speed turns and (2) leaning the bike and your body to negotiate faster turns. The faster that you go, the more that leaning (or angulation) comes into play. Turning the handlebar at higher speeds will only cause the front wheel to plow or wash out.

Most slow-speed turning techniques are really balancing techniques. Now, it's time to raise the ante. Going faster doesn't mean riding recklessly or dangerously if you understand the techniques, take time to practice them, and don't let your speed increase at a faster rate than your skill and confidence.

107

Speed Thrills

Regardless of the technique that you plan to use for a given turn, it's crucial to determine how much speed you can carry into it. If you need to slow down, there's one rule you should never violate: Do your hard braking before you enter, so the wheels are free to roll once turning begins.

The best line is the same one you use on a road bike or when driving: Set up wide, cut through the apex, then exit to the outside edge. Think of it as trying to straighten the turn by making it as shallow as possible. This is the way to carry maximum speed. You can't always follow this ideal line on a technical trail, but always look for the opportunity. Realize, though, that there may be drastic changes in traction in different areas of a turn. When this is the case, the fastest line may not be the straightest one.

Practicing fast turns is lots of fun. In fact, it's downright exhilarating.

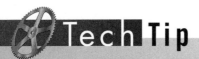

Your tires can have a dramatically positive or negative effect on your ability to negotiate high-speed turns. Performance depends on such key tire characteristics as width, profile, tread pattern, and knob size, plus the amount of air pressure that you run.

As you practice turning techniques and drills, you might begin to think that your tires are inhibiting your ability. It could be true if, for instance, you're riding muddy trails on tires designed for dry, hard-packed conditions. But before you switch, I encourage you to do the following experiment to make sure the rubber is really the reason.

Make several trial runs through turns on your current tires, then ride exactly the same course on the tires that you're thinking about switching to. Be absolutely certain that the front tires have identical air pressure and that the rear tires do as well. These should be the pressures that you've found to be the best suited to your weight, terrain, and riding style.

Too often, riders are quick to judge tires without an objective comparison. Do everything you can to isolate tire performance from the other variables. If you do see advantages to switching, start using the new tires for all rides, not just for races. That's the only way you can learn the fine points of their traction and handling.

For me, one of the biggest excitements in mountain biking comes when my tires are no longer firmly connected to the ground, when my direction is controlled only by weight shifts and steering inputs. Feeling comfortable with wheel drift is absolutely the key to going fast, and the only way to get comfortable is with plenty of practice.

Locate a dirt-road loop with a smooth surface that you can ride over and over, making left turns and right turns. Before practicing, install the tires you ride or race on most often. Tire treads can make a big difference in turning traction and all-around bike behavior. For instance, when you start to drift in a dry, hard-packed turn on knobs that are tall and soft, the tire may squirm and slide suddenly as the knobs fold over. If you're not used to this feedback, it's a big problem. Also, always inflate the tires to your optimum air pressure. I'm a firm believer in training at the same air pressure at which you race. Otherwise, you'll never quite learn the limits of traction or the fine points of bike control.

A difference of 10 psi (from, say, 25 to 35 psi) can completely change a tire's behavior. Less than 30 psi is apt to make a tire squirmy and unpredictable. Between 30 and 40 psi is comfortable and the tire will corner well, but depending on your weight, it may not be enough to prevent pinch flats on rocky ground. Harder tires drift a little quicker in turns, but I'm willing to accept this to get maximum pinch-flat protection. It's not a problem if you learn how to deal with firm inflation during practice.

Body-angulation turn. This basic turn is made while coasting. Hold the crankarms horizontal and angle your upper body at the hips toward the outside of the turn. The bike stays relatively upright unless you have a berm to angle it into. Use a body-angulation turn when speed is fairly slow and stability and traction are not in question. It's also best for rough terrain when you have to be out of the saddle to absorb shock with your legs. Also use it for banked turns or turns with good traction where you can simply lean to strike a balance among centrifugal force, gravity, and traction. At higher speeds, though, on a slippery surface with no berm to help hold your wheels in, you'll feel unstable with the crankarms horizontal. It'll feel as though the tires want to slide to the outside.

Traction determines how much speed you can carry through a turn and how much body English you need to keep the tires biting. Angulation helps improve traction because leaning your upper body to the outside of the turn puts weight over each tire's contact patch (the section in contact with the ground). For instance, as the bike leans to the left, you lean to the right.

Step hard on the outside pedal and use upper-body angulation to keep the wheels pinned to the ground.

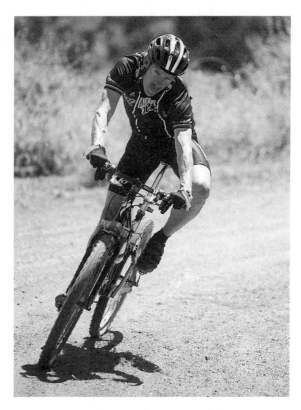

Your weight drives the knobs into the dirt, lessening the negative aspects of centrifugal force and keeping more tread on the trail.

Weighted-pedal turn. This is the technique for higher speeds or when the surface is slippery. It lets you use your body weight to increase turning traction.

As you enter the turn, put your outside foot at the bottom of its pedal stroke. Press hard and hold it there. Angle your upper body toward the outside of the turn (as in the body-angulation turn). By standing on the outside pedal, you increase traction by concentrating your weight on each tire's contact patch. You also lower your center of gravity by moving your weight to the lowest possible place on the bike (the pedal at its lowest point). In this way, you can ride tight turns at a higher speed. The key as speed increases is to tilt your hips with the bike to the inside of the turn, but angulate to keep your shoulders over your outside foot and your weight focused on the pedal. Try putting slightly more weight on the front wheel by pressing down on the outside handlebar grip. This improves front-tire traction.

Making a successful fast turn depends on finding the balance between leaning the bike and keeping enough weight on the tires to prevent them from sliding out. It means a lot of side-to-side weighting. Some of this is done with your hands, not just your feet. Subtle shifts in your weight or center of gravity can help your stability. Experience is the best teacher.

Some riders like to point their inside knees into the turn as they stand hard on the outside pedals. Try this and see how it accentuates the turning forces. In some situations, this also helps your balance by giving you a wider stance. Pointing the knee has fallen out of favor among some roadies who specialize in criteriums, which have dozens of fast 90-degree turns. These racers claim that an extended knee acts like an air brake and slows them unnecessarily. This isn't a factor in trail riding, but better balance often is. Practice pointing your knee so this technique will be in your arsenal.

Outrigger turn. When you go fast through turns, your wheels are likely to drift a bit, that is, slide toward the outside. Usually, you don't want this to happen, but the faster you go, the stronger the centrifugal force pulls you

Use your inside leg like an outrigger to catch yourself if the wheels slide out.

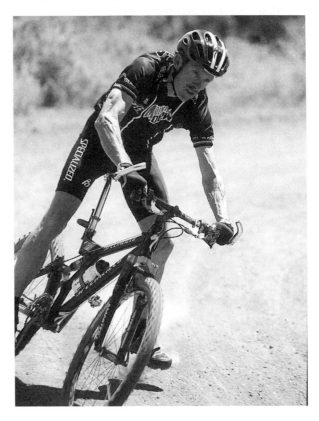

to the outside of the turn. You need to get comfortable with wheel drift so you don't overreact and crash. Learn to relax and enjoy this cheap thrill.

The trick when going through a fast, slippery turn is to take your inside foot off its pedal and hold it near the ground. This separates your legs to give you a wider stance. It increases stability and improves your ability to balance. It's comparable to the balance you gain by sticking out your arms when walking along a log. Plus, if the rear wheel slides out, you can use your leg as an outrigger to prevent a fall.

This technique works best with the saddle braced against the thigh of your outside leg. Hold your inside leg to the side, knee slightly bent and toes pointed up, with your foot just above the ground. Then you're ready to tap the ground to stay upright.

It's surprising how far you can drift without actually sliding out, so hang tough as you learn. Don't be too quick to touch the ground.

Off-camber turn. This is a tough one when you're moving fast. You come whipping into a turn and . . . there's nothing there—no berm to ride against. The trail just falls away toward the outside. In this situation (or whenever the terrain drops off), use extreme angulation and weight the outside pedal like I've just described to keep the tires sticking to the trail.

Off-camber turns are very sensitive to braking forces. It's critical to recognize these turns and reduce your speed before you start cornering. You

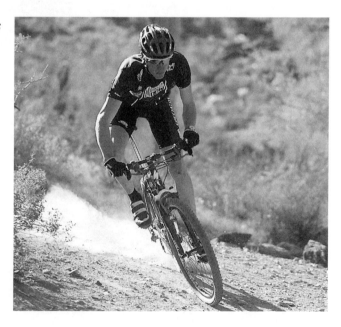

If the rear wheel starts to slide, countersteer with the front wheel.

may want to take your inside foot off the pedal because once your tires start to slide, the missing camber just lets them go. With your outrigger ready, you can exaggerate your turning technique as much as necessary to find traction and stability.

Countersteering. In any type of turn, if the rear wheel does break loose, regain control by countersteering with the front wheel—turning it in the same direction that the rear wheel is sliding. In other words, turn the front wheel toward the outside of the turn. It's similar to the reaction you should have when your car is sliding on an icy road. Countersteering with the front end controls how fast and far the rear end will slide.

Lots of times, you'll have varying amounts of traction through a turn. You'll sense wheel drift and know that your line is changing. To keep your tires biting, you need to make rapid but subtle adjustments to your body position and steering. You always have a choice—you can either let the laws of physics decide your fate or you can take control.

Countersteering is another of the many things that pro racer John Tomac is great at. For him, it's totally instinctive. If his rear wheel starts to slide out, he stays relaxed. He countersteers into the skid while counter-balancing his weight. This lets him regain traction and pull the bike more upright to get his weight back on top. Then he exits the turn with no loss of momentum. I've seen him do it a thousand times.

Square turn. When you're on a dirt road and don't have to worry about damaging the terrain, learn the technique of "squaring off" a turn. This term describes how your line goes from straight to a sharp turn to straight again in a different direction. By pivoting your rear wheel around the radius of the turn, you can change your line almost instantly. Coast, get your weight slightly forward, begin to turn left or right, then snatch the rear brake to initiate a rear-wheel slide. The back of the bike pivots to the side to create the turn. Adjust the amount of slide with countersteer like I just described above. Countersteer more (toward the outside of the turn) to lessen the slide, or keep your front wheel straight ahead to continue the slide or slide faster. Let go of the rear brake as soon as you've turned enough, so you won't kill your momentum.

For safety while learning, put out your inside foot to catch yourself if you overdo it and begin to slide out completely. Once you get the hang of squaring off a turn, you'll be able to do it with both feet on the pedals. Remember, this is not a trail-friendly technique, so use it only on dirt roads or in areas where it won't accelerate trail erosion.

Brake Not

Your tires will be at the edge of their traction in the apex of a high-speed turn. If they start to slide and you panic and snatch the brakes, you'll slide out and probably go down. The alternative if you really need to slow down is to sit upright and grab the rear brake only. You'll still slide out, but it will be more controlled. If you grab the front brake instead, you're a goner.

The proper technique is to slow to the correct speed before turning begins. Look for a relatively smooth patch of ground with good traction. Use it to brake as hard as necessary, then enter the turn with your wheels rolling free.

To reduce the chance of inadvertent braking while in a tricky turn, try a technique that works well for me. I extend my fingers so they're not resting on the brake levers—especially the lever that's hooked to the front brake. You'll notice a big improvement in turning traction when you're not unconsciously feathering the brakes.

Experiment, comparing different kinds of turns and techniques. Practice all the methods I've described. Practice turns to the left, to the right, and on snaking trails with quick direction changes. You'll find that different turning techniques work better for different surfaces, speeds, and radii. To ride like a champion, you need to be adept at every combination. You can't practice too much, and I guarantee that you will never stop learning.

16 Switchbacks

A Tough Test
of Balance and Control

The question that people ask me most often is how to ride switchbacks. And they ask for a very good reason. Whether it's on a climb or a descent, a switchback requires a delicate mixture of speed, balance, traction, and steering control. The consequences of a mistake range from the frustration of having to dismount and walk, to slipping over the edge into some bottomless chasm.

Switchbacks, which are turns sharper than 90 degrees on hillsides, differ from other turns because you ride so slowly. It's simply impossible to carry speed when the trail nearly doubles back on itself. If you have trouble riding switchbacks, it's probably because you have difficulty balancing at slow speed. Your wheels' helpful gyroscopic effect is missing. Simply trying to stay upright keeps you from concentrating on the mechanics of the turn.

But there's another problem: the repercussions of screwing up. By their nature, switchbacks are in steep terrain. Often, one side of the trail isn't there—it borders on a precipice, leaving little room for error. I remember a ride on the Colorado Trail with Team GT rider Greg Randolph. We came to a pretty technical switchback—there was even a stream cutting through it—and Greg hit a rock that was under the water. In a blink, he fell over the edge. He didn't go very far into the air, but it was so steep that he tumbled

35 feet before stopping. He owed all those cuts and bruises to the risks inherent in switchbacks. They can snag even the best rider.

So, yes, you must be wary of the difficulties that switchbacks present, but you don't have to fear them. You can learn to ride switchbacks well. The alternatives—stalling on uphills or losing control going down—are a major source of frustration and a frequent cause of crashes. In races, the ability to ride switchbacks can separate the winner from the losers in the closing laps. When fatigue sets in, the skilled riders stay on their bikes while the others crash or walk.

A Matter of Balance

The trackstand and balancing skills discussed in chapter 2 are the same skills you need to ride a switchback's slow hairpin turn. But in terms of cornering technique, you need not follow the basic rule of starting wide, cutting through the apex, then emerging wide. The reason that you do this in a corner that is not a switchback is to straighten it as much as possible so you can keep your speed. You have a different priority in switchbacks, however. It's not speed you're concerned with, it's momentum.

Often, the apex of a switchback turn is the steepest part. Your chances of keeping the bike rolling improve a lot if you can make the turn shallower. On climbs, this has the added benefit of conserving muscle energy. During recreational rides, you can simply take the widest line all the way around the switchback to reduce the pitch to its minimum. During races, you can fudge, cutting corners either uphill or downhill where you can save time without breaking traction, blowing momentum, or losing control.

Avoid approaching a switchback on an inside line. The turn then becomes so tight and steep that chances for success are slim. When you're climbing, the pitch may be so vertical that it's simply impossible to ride. You're then at risk because it's very hard to dismount in the middle of a switchback without stumbling back down the hill. When you're descending, the apex may be so sheer that you're gripped by the fear of falling over the handlebar. Part of smart switchback riding is planning ahead to avoid emergencies like these—and always having a bail-out plan in case you goof.

Going Up

When tackling an uphill switchback, match your speed to the tightness of the switchback. This will be in small increments, of course, because

A great way to get the hang of riding through slow, tight turns is to ride in circles. You can practice this in your driveway or yard.

The challenge is to make the circle as small as possible. This requires riding very slowly and using the brakes. The handlebar will be turned so much that you can't make full pedal strokes because your knees will hit it. The solution is to ratchet the pedals, making partial strokes. Do this smoothly and gently because too much force will push the front wheel and widen the circle. It takes lots of balance to turn this tight. At times, you'll be almost at a trackstand. Go clockwise. Go counter-clockwise. Learn to make a smooth, tight transition from one direction to the other.

Even though I've been riding for many years, I still practice this simple drill. In winter, for instance, I back the cars out into the snow and ride laps in the garage with my son, Rhyler, who rides his BMX bike. We set up an obstacle course and chase each other. We make a contest of seeing who can turn the tightest. It's fun, and it definitely translates to the trail.

you're climbing. Too much speed, and you can't turn as sharply. Less speed than the turn can handle may cause you to stall if your rear wheel hits something or loses traction.

Riding uphill switchbacks combines principles discussed in chapter 13—such as shifting your body weight to maintain traction—with the balance required for a slow tight-radius turn. Shift gears as necessary to keep pedaling in the hardest sections. This is where a smooth, round pedal stroke really pays off. Choppy power pulses are likely to break rear-wheel traction in steep uphill turns.

To enhance traction as a switchback's radius narrows, position your hips toward the outside of the turn. You can make this happen simply by leaning your head and shoulders inside. When you do it right, your spine curves in the same direction as the turn. Next, pivot your neck so you can see the trail ahead.

Concentrate on your line. Look for the widest, easiest route, taking into account roots, rocks, and the need for adequate traction. Lots of riders forget this visual discipline. If you look directly in front of your wheel, you won't be thinking far enough ahead to plan for obstacles by adjusting steering and body posture.

As your ability improves, try the advanced technique of popping a wheelie to adjust your direction. This is an easy trick on a steep climb. Do it by pulling up the front wheel a few inches as you apply downward pressure on the pedals. Then set the wheel down to one side and continue your

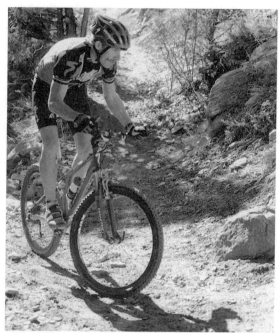

When climbing a switchback, approach wide to open the turning radius and lessen the grade (top). *Good slow-speed balance and climbing skills let you concentrate on your line* (bottom), *rather than worry about staying upright and maintaining traction.*

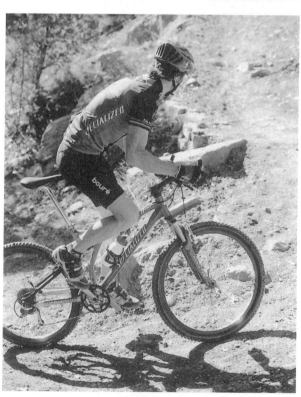

smooth pedaling. This can change your line by several inches, which may be just enough to miss an object or reduce the grade to find better traction.

If you sense that a switchback is not going to be ridable, don't wait too long to dismount. Do it while you're still in balance and have control of your bike and body. This will prevent the most common cause of bad falls—tipping toward the downhill side. When you tip, you can't put a foot down to hold yourself up, because your foot won't reach the ground when your other leg is still over the bike. You go over and your bike follows on top. It can be a messy tumble. Get off on the uphill side while you're still in control.

Coming Down

Downhill switchbacks combine tight slow-speed turns with the additional challenge of precise braking. In fact, the main reason that downhill switchbacks are so intimidating is because the steepness requires downhill braking even while turning. This tests all of your balancing, turning, and braking skills at the same time.

The secret to maximum control is to keep your bike nearly vertical. Remember, at slow speeds you can do this while turning, because you don't have any centrifugal force to counteract. Slow down before sharp turning starts, so you won't have to squeeze the brakes as hard when you're steering. Ideally, choose a line that has smooth places for braking traction. As always, stay off the front brake when the handlebar is turned on wet, slippery rocks and roots.

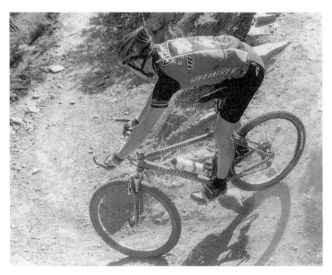

When descending a switchback, use an outside-inside-outside line. Approach wide, cut directly through the apex, then exit wide. This reduces turning time and provides more chances to brake.

As opposed to when you're climbing a switchback and seeking a shallower, easier, outside line, you can choose to cut through the apex when going downhill. This requires less turning but it steepens the drop, so control your speed going in. Don't forget that your speed must allow you to turn even more to exit the switchback (and there's likely to be something really unpleasant waiting if you miscalculate and go over the edge). The good news is that taking a straighter line through the apex gives you a chance to brake. You transform the switchback's big curve into two turns—one that starts wide at the top, then one that exits wide at the bottom, with a relatively straight drop between. Go through in a gear that's big enough to give you more exit speed if you want it.

Especially in a downhill switchback, always remember: Look where you want your wheels to go, not where you're afraid they'll end up. I can give you plenty of examples to drive home this point, but this one should do.

The race was on the Hermosa Creek Trail, a supertechnical, 20-mile-long singletrack near Durango, Colorado. In the direction we were going, there was a major drop-off on the left side. I was behind a top rider, Mike Kloser from Vail, Colorado, also known as Alpine Eddie. He went into a sharp turn a little too hot and felt the danger. Despite his years of experience, he glanced into the ravine. Over he went. He actually rode part of the way down before bailing out. His bike went cartwheeling. He was so far down—I couldn't believe it. I also was amazed that he didn't get hurt. It took him a long time to climb out of there, giving me the chance to build a nice lead.

Remember this crash when descending steep switchbacks. You're probably going to be just inches from the trail edge and some very nasty stuff. Don't look. Don't be intimidated. Keep your focus on the line that you want to take. The more relaxed you feel, the better focus you will have. Relaxation comes from confidence, and confidence comes from practice. It's amazing the difference that strong focus makes.

The risk of inadvertent nose wheelies is always present during slow, steep downhill turns, so keep your weight low and rearward. On some switchbacks, your butt may be so far over the back wheel that your chest is above the saddle.

Sometimes, though, a nose wheelie can be good. It can help you correct a dangerous line. When your butt is off the rear of the saddle and you're using the front brake, it's easy to slide the rear wheel several inches to the side. You don't have to actually lift it into the air—in fact, that's risky on a steep descent. Just use your hips to twitch the bike. There's so little weight on the rear wheel that it will slip right over.

This move accomplishes the same thing as squaring off a turn (see chapter 15 for that technique), but it's not as damaging to the trail. Remember, avoid riding in ways that could accelerate erosion. Skidding is okay on dirt roads, but not on singletrack unless you're having a true emergency. By the way, locking up your wheels because you're recklessly riding too fast is not the kind of emergency that I mean.

Releasing Your Feet

Even the best riders sometimes need to dismount in a switchback. In a race, for instance, a switchback that guys can handle during the early laps may become too tough to ride when fatigue takes over. Or a guy may wad it up in front of you, leaving you with nothing to do but stop. So part of switchback skill is being able to get out of the pedals cleanly to avoid crashing.

I've seen lots of riders struggle with this. A rider may concentrate so much on climbing traction, applying power, turning, and balancing that he doesn't have time to put a foot down when he loses it. Or, he unthinkingly puts his favorite foot down—most riders have a strong preference for either their left or right—and it happens to be the one on the downhill side. So long.

I'm a right-footer, and I like to get my foot out at the bottom of the stroke. I could be in trouble if I need to pull a foot to prevent a fall while my right foot is both at the top of the stroke and on the downhill side. Fortunately, I've practiced left-foot releases. It still isn't instinctive, but by balancing for a second, I can make the correct choice. This is yet another instance where the ability to do a trackstand or stay upright at creeping speed pays off. It gives you a second to think.

Practice releases when you practice trackstands. Release with each foot, clicking out at every position of the pedal circle. You'll find spots where this feels pretty awkward, but that's the point. Get used to doing it in safe situations so your ability will be better in dangerous ones.

Remember that the easiest motion with the least restraint will be when your foot pivot is parallel to the pedal, as opposed to an upward pull while trying to twist out. If you're still having release problems, you may need to lube the pedal's mechanism or lighten its spring setting. Replacing old worn cleats also makes release easier and more consistent.

As you practice releases, practice clipping in. The goal here is to develop the ability to find and engage the pedals without looking down. This can spare you big problems on the trail, where diverting your eyes downward

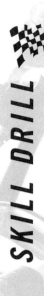

Even a small obstacle can pose big problems in a switchback. Your front wheel may make it safely past, then the rear may strike the obstacle and kill your momentum. You're forced to put a foot down to keep from toppling over. Next comes the difficulty of starting up again.

Spare yourself this frustration. Here's a slow-speed maneuvering drill to learn how the rear wheel tracks through a tight turn in relation to the front. You can do this on flat ground. Set down a line of a dozen stones (or paper cups) several feet apart. Weave through these stones as if you're riding a slalom course.

First, try to pass each stone so it's on the same side of your wheels. To do this without running over the stone with your rear wheel, you'll need to make a fairly wide arc and wait a bit longer before turning back in the other direction.

Next, try to pass each stone so your front wheel is on its outside but your rear wheel is on the inside. This requires a shallower arc and quicker turning.

Soon, you'll know where your rear wheel is in relation to any object you pass with the front. This awareness needs to become second nature. When it is, you'll be much better at negotiating switchbacks in the real world of ruts, rocks, and roots.

for even a nanosecond can send you off-line. More than one tree has been debarked due to such a mistake.

Remounting

If you come off the bike on an uphill switchback or on the steeper sections going downhill, don't try to remount. It's too difficult to get going again with that much gravity involved. Instead, walk or run to the top of the climb or to a shallower section of the descent. In a race, watch out for other riders coming through. They're at their limits of control. Stay out of the riding line until you're back on your bike.

Before remounting, make sure you're in the right gear. If you stalled on a climb and need to start in an easier gear, hand shift to a larger cog. Grab the pedal with your hand and turn the crankarm while you're pushing the bike to a good place to get back on.

Remounting is something else you should practice, especially if you're a racer. You can save a few seconds if you develop an efficient technique. Some riders like to leap onto the bike (if they still have enough energy), then get into the pedals and go. They take the saddle's impact with the inner thigh of their left leg when remounting from the right, or vice versa. This is how cyclocross racers do it.

Another method that some riders use works like a skateboard push-off. Let's say you're remounting from the right side. Clip your right foot in, push off once or twice with your left foot to get rolling, then swing your left leg over to mount the bike. You can switch sides and feet depending on your preference and the conditions. This method can work on smooth flats or slight downhills, but it doesn't produce enough momentum on uphills or when trail conditions are rough or soft. There's too much rolling resistance. Also, be careful in wet conditions because your push-off foot may slip and cause an awkward fall.

Often, it's most efficient simply to stand on the uphill side, swing your leg over, clip in, pull the pedal up, push it down as you move onto the saddle, then clip in with the other foot. The quicker your second foot connects, the better, but sometimes you may need to pedal several revolutions to build momentum before you can engage it. This is often the case on uphill restarts, where you need to keep the front wheel down as you begin applying rear-wheel power.

Remember to keep your chest low and pull back on the handlebar, not up. It's another instance where good balance pays off. You don't have to pedal frantically and steer wildly to stay upright if you've developed the ability to calmly focus on control and traction at slow speed.

On a downhill, get the crankarms horizontal right away. This should be your first priority, even ahead of clipping in. You can't absorb bumps or brake with the crankarms vertical. Assume the low, off-saddle attack position, with flexed arms and knees. Here's where it's important to have shoes with rubber soles that won't slip off the pedals. You can coast downhill in this position with the pedal under the arch of your foot, waiting for a good moment to engage the cleat. Be sure to keep your weight back, especially when you don't have the security of being clipped in.

17 Drop-Offs and Ledges

Fighting the Fear Factor

A drop-off and a ledge are actually the same thing—an abrupt mini-cliff across the trail. The reason I use both terms is to distinguish the one that juts up in front of you (ledge) from the one that disappears from under you (drop-off). With this in mind, how do you transform a drop-off into a ledge, or vice versa? Just turn around and ride toward it from the opposite direction.

Even if the trail is essentially flat, think of riding a drop-off as a downhill technique and of riding a ledge as an uphill technique. The goal is to get over these obstacles with enough dexterity to keep your momentum and control.

Relaxation is probably the greatest aid to making the right moves. Most riders tense up and clamp death grips on their handlebars when facing an abrupt mini-wall or looking over a scary-but-ridable cliff. I'm not denying that these can be anxious moments, but you must fight this fear, which stiffens your whole body and makes fluid position changes and balance corrections impossible. Relaxation will come naturally as you practice the following techniques, develop your skill, and gain confidence.

There are two distinct ways to ride drop-offs, depending on your speed. The first is when you attempt to go over without slowing. This is certainly the preferred method in a race because it preserves momentum.

Drop-offs are intimidating because the front wheel is about to plunge straight down and it seems like you'll pivot over the handlebar. The potential is certainly there, so you're right to have a healthy amount of appre-

125

TRUE STORY

Some drop-offs are so hairy that they scare even the best riders. A great example is called Bailey's Bailout, a frightening feature of the 1994 world championship course in Vail, Colorado.

Bailey's Bailout is a series of several drop-offs. Or you might just call it a rocky cliff. It has a total height of about 20 feet. The approach is blind—you can't see down this section until you're right at the top—and it's made even more treacherous by loose, slippery dirt. I knew I could ride this nightmare because I'd done it in previous races. But it always put me right at the edge of survival.

At the world championship, most of the men, myself included, decided to jump off on each lap through Bailey's Bailout. We half-walked, half-slid to the bottom. I saw two riders in front of me break bones when they attempted to ride it and crashed heavily. It was that hazardous.

Now guess what happened in the women's race. Several of them rode the thing with less difficulty than it took the guys to walk it. That's an impressive testament to the skill that's engendered by finesse and relaxation. Mountain biking is often thought of as a power sport. There's much more to it, as women prove all the time.

hension. Although correct technique will do a lot to minimize the risks, don't forget that dismounting and walking is always an option. I don't mind admitting that sometimes that's what I do. It's better to lose a little time being cautious than a lot of time untangling yourself from a crash. That said, most people can ride bigger drop-offs than they think they can, even at faster speeds. Don't sell yourself short—practice.

Beyond a certain height, a drop-off (or a ledge) ridden at slow speed will hit your large chainring. This distance can vary by an inch or two, depending on bottom bracket height and other factors, but the result is always the same—chainring damage followed by a crash. With experience, you'll become a pretty good judge of what your bike can clear. When in doubt, play it safe like I do, dismount, and walk the bike across the obstacle. If the chainring clears, you have the option of going back to try to ride it.

Drop Offs at Fast Speeds

You're most likely to encounter drop-offs on descents, which means you'll approach them at relatively high speed. For this discussion, let's say that the one you're coming to is about 18 inches deep. That's enough to look scary. It's pretty typical of what you'll find when riding fun, technical singletrack. Trails in the Rocky Mountains and Utah have plenty of drop-offs this size.

First, check the situation on the other side of the drop-off. Your objective is to stay off the brakes and keep your speed, so you want the trail on the far side to be clear—nothing dangerous waiting for your wheels and no quick turn to make. If that's the case, you can ride right over the drop-off. You're not actually jumping and trying to create air time, but you'll get some. How much depends on your launch speed.

As you reach the lip, be in the attack position, crouched low over the saddle with your arms and knees flexed. When you land, you must be off the saddle to use your legs as shock absorbers. Keep the crankarms horizontal and your weight centered or slightly back, never forward. The steeper the descent, the farther back you need to be.

Stay aware of the front wheel. You may need to lift it a bit to ensure that you touch down on the rear wheel first or on both wheels simultaneously. Try to avoid landing on the front wheel first or you could lose control. It's easy to swerve or tip forward, especially on longer flights from bigger drop-offs. Just as important, you must be off the brakes. Upon landing, if your wheels aren't free to roll, your body could be thrown forward—maybe even over the handlebar.

For drop-offs at faster speeds, center your weight over the saddle and loft the front wheel enough to land on both wheels together or the rear wheel first.

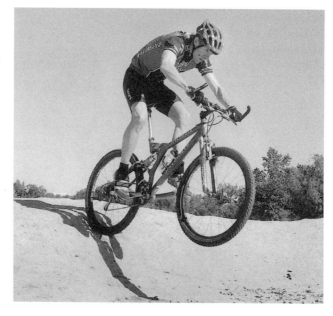

For most riders, the fear of crashing is a huge impediment to riding drop-offs at faster speeds. The best way to overcome it is to build your skill systematically. Start practicing by riding off a curb onto smooth pavement. Always wear your helmet and gloves. Go over fast enough to catch some air and land on both wheels together. If your front wheel touchs down first, practice lifting it a bit at the takeoff—just enough to keep the bike parallel to the landing surface. As you gain more confidence, graduate to small drop-offs on trails. Keep building up until an 18-incher feels as easy as a curb.

Drop-Offs at Slow Speeds

If you arrive at the drop-off at slow speed or need to brake because there's a challenge on the other side—an immediate sharp turn, for instance—this calls for an entirely different technique. Now, you go over the drop-off at walking speed, getting no air at all.

First, adjust your line so you approach and go over the drop-off perpendicular to the edge (or as close to perpendicular as possible). If you're not perpendicular, it could make the landing and runout more difficult because you may not be able to correct your line before you reach a turn or obstacle.

The next key is body position. You must have your weight way back so

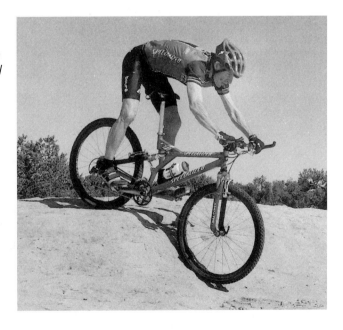

On a slow-speed drop-off, move your weight way back to prevent an endo as the front wheel goes down.

the front wheel doesn't stop at the bottom and pitch you over. Push the handlebar forward as you drop the front wheel down. Your chest will be so far back and so low that it might touch the saddle. Your goal is to make the bike smoothly follow the contour of the drop-off. As the front wheel lands and rolls, bring your weight to the center again to help the rear wheel drop. You can then resume your normal riding position.

When you do it right, it's a flowing motion, like water cascading over rocks in a stream. The shift in body weight protects each wheel from a hard, jarring, control-threatening impact. During practice, you may want to lower the saddle so your body has more freedom to move. Raise it back to regular height as your skill improves.

All hard braking must be done on the approach or after both wheels are past the drop-off. As you go over, release the front brake lever and be careful not to accidentally snatch it when the front wheel hits—the perfect setup for an endo. Stay off the front brake until the drop-off is behind you and the wheel is rolling enough to establish traction. In technical sections, you may be close to a trackstand at the top or bottom of a drop-off, so it pays to review the balancing techniques described in chapter 2.

Start practicing on flat ground by getting in and out of the extreme rearward body position—butt over the rear wheel, chest on the saddle. Ride slow, coast, and make this move with the crankarms horizontal. Again, it'll probably help a lot to lower the saddle. Once you're smooth and comfortable, go to a tall curb to combine this move with a slow approach and the effects of dropping over. When you're ready, graduate to an actual drop-off that has a steep side but curved runout to help your front wheel make the transition from downward to forward. This is a safer place for learning technique than a drop-off with a sharp 90-degree angle at the bottom.

Ledges

Let's turn and ride back up this trail. Now that 18-inch drop-off looms as a ledge. To get up and over, you need to perform one essential move—a power-stroke wheelie (for more information, see chapter 12). But there are other requirements as well. Climbing ledges takes finesse, not just strength.

First, how is your fitness? You're most likely to encounter ledges on a climb. If you're already pushing hard and breathing like the old Iron Horse steam engine that runs between the Colorado towns of Durango and Silverton, you may not have enough juice left to do a wheelie. You need to work on your fitness if proper technique isn't enough to get you over ledges.

Arrive at the ledge with good momentum, then try to retain it. Make your power-stroke wheelie with enough force to take the front wheel up and set it on top of the ledge. You want to avoid any head-on contact that'll stop you dead. Then instantly surge your weight toward the front. The taller the ledge, the more force you must put into this move. Consider how much you weigh compared to your 25-pound bike. The bike will go where your weight takes it.

In addition to providing momentum, this forward surge lightens the rear wheel. Now, you're at the critical point. You have to stop your legs for a second with the crankarms horizontal to prevent slamming a pedal into the ledge. Resume pedaling just as the rear tire makes contact. Apply enough power to make the tire bite and roll up but not so much that it slips, spins out, and stops you instantly. Your technique is perfect when the rear wheel rolls up so smoothly that you barely feel an impact.

To scale a ledge, start with a power-stroke wheelie that's strong enough to set the front wheel on top (top). Then immediately shift your weight forward to take the rear wheel up (bottom). Resume pedaling as soon as there is clearance.

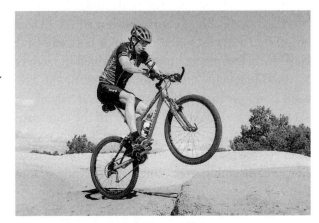

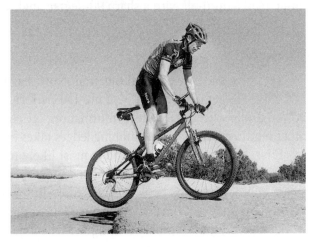

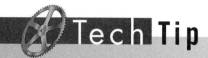

Tech Tip

When riding over tall objects, you run the risk of bashing your large chainring. You can do this without too much problem when the obstacle is relatively compliant, like a log. But ledges and drop-offs are never forgiving. When a chainring's aluminum teeth bite into rock, the damage may be so bad that you'll be limited to your small chainrings for the rest of the ride.

At $30 or more per chainring, this is an expensive mistake. For about the same price, you can buy a chainring protector. This metal protector bolts on like a fourth chainring, but it has no teeth. It's slightly larger in diameter than your big ring so it takes the impact of a too-tall obstacle. This lets you ride with more freedom. You don't have to stop and walk for fear that a ledge or drop-off is a bit too big. Most shops carry chainring protectors or can order one for you.

As always in slow-speed maneuvers, good balance is essential. It's what enables you to lose some momentum in a precarious position yet not have to turn all your attention to staying upright. It lets you concentrate instead on the moves you need to make. If you do stall halfway over a ledge, good balance keeps you in control so you can pull a foot and prevent a fall. It gives you confidence that makes riding ledges a lot easier. Practice your trackstands and slow-speed drills.

18 Crashing

The Right Instincts
Reduce the Damage

Crashing is funny, sort of. At least, it gives us a few entertaining phrases. Can you imagine what it looks like when a rider "wads it up" or "augers in" or does a "pile driver"? Then there's the "yard sale," where a guy leaves stuff strewn along the trail. You find what's left of him by following the debris. Sooner or later, each of us will blast into a turn too fast and "throw it all away." Even more vivid is the image of a "rag doll"—an out-of-control rider flopping on the ground with legs and arms in every direction.

When you crash—and you surely will—the right reaction can go a long way toward keeping that smile on your face. I know riders who crash a lot without getting hurt and riders who crash infrequently but suffer relatively severe injuries. Your chances of coming away from a crash unscathed are much better if you know how to fall.

Tuck and Roll

A few years ago, I attended a cycling camp that featured a coach from Poland. He taught me how to react whenever I find myself in one of cycling's most dangerous predicaments—an unexpected head-first dismount over the front of the bike. Almost always, the best response is what is called

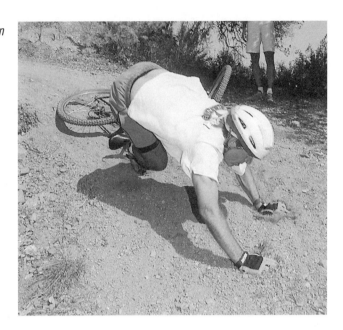

Here's why crashing can crack a collarbone and why your hands will take a beating if you don't wear gloves. It's instinctive to break a fall with outstretched arms, but the impact goes straight to your shoulders if you don't dissipate it by tucking and rolling.

the tuck-and-roll technique. This applies to road riders as well as to mountain bikers.

To learn how to tuck and roll, we went to a gym and used the tumbling mats. It's actually an easy drill: Run and dive forward. Break your fall by first contacting the mat with your hands, then immediately absorb the impact by bending your wrists and elbows as you tuck your head and the shoulder that's closest to the mat. Roll across that shoulder and your back. The key is to let your arms collapse under the impact to dissipate the force. The rolling motion serves the same purpose. In a real crash, if you stick into the ground like a javelin, the impact goes directly into your body, making serious damage more likely.

The goal is to make a tuck and roll instinctive during an actual crash. Practice the above drill on mats or soft grass until it becomes easy and ingrained. Refresh your instincts with practice once in awhile. Become adept at rolling over each shoulder because you won't always get a chance to use your favorite side out on the trail.

This technique can spare you from a broken collarbone, probably the most common serious injury in cycling. It's often caused by landing on a rigid, outstretched arm. Force is transmitted straight to your shoulder girdle and your collarbone snaps. In general, the more relaxed your body is during a crash, the less damage you will suffer. Think "shock absorber."

If you've never tumbled, begin practicing from your knees and roll forward. Once you have the hang of it, try it from a standing position. After that, try it from a walk and next a jog with a little dive. Work your way up to a running tumble.

If you can't catch on, you may be too inflexible. Consider a stretching program, which in itself can safeguard muscles and joints when you're flailing around in a crash. I believe that flexibility can even prevent crashes. When you can move fluidly all around the bike with a full range of motion, you can make more of the position adjustments that keep you upright.

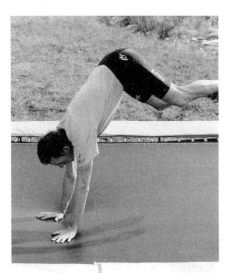

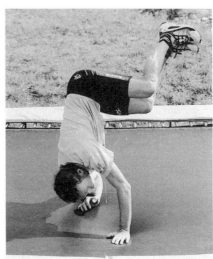

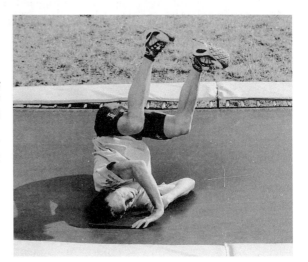

Practice this tuck-and-roll drill to develop the right instincts in a crash. Stop your fall with outstretched arms (top left), *but when your hands touch the ground, immediately collapse your elbows and dip a shoulder* (top right). *By rolling across your shoulder and back* (bottom), *you dissipate energy. You can also see the value of wearing gloves and a helmet while riding.*

Ned's KNOWLEDGE

I don't know many riders who stretch, even though flexibility has obvious benefits during crashes (and may even help prevent them). The most common excuse that I hear is, "I don't have time." Well, I don't buy it. I used to say the same thing until I found an easy way to fit a few minutes of stretching into nearly every day.

I've become a TV stretcher. Instead of just sitting there watching a program, I get on the floor and work on my flexibility. It doesn't feel like a chore, because I'm barely thinking about it. My focus is on the show. My technique is to stretch slowly to the point where I feel the pull, hold for 15 to 20 seconds, back off gently, then repeat. After doing each stretch a couple of times, I move on unless I sense some tightness that needs extra work. I keep it casual, not regimented.

Usually I do this routine in the evening, which ensures that my body is already pretty loose from a full day of regular activities and my ride. I recommend this time of day as opposed to first thing in the morning, when your body is tighter. I do a little stretching after rising, to get the kinks out, but it's better to be warmed up when trying to improve flexibility. For expert guidance, I recommend Bob Anderson's classic book, *Stretching*. It specifies all the best stretches for cyclists.

Before a race, I ride a little to warm up, then stretch to loosen my muscles and tendons. I want to free their range of motion. This is important because flexibility pays off in better bike control, and supple muscles are more efficient at turning the crankarms. It could also spare me from a muscle pull or joint injury in a crash.

Now that I'm over 40, I think stretching is more important than ever. Looking back at my cycling career, probably 95 percent of my injuries have been the result of what I call overuse, which relates directly to muscle strains and pulls caused by inflexibility. Younger guys can ride right through a muscle pull; older guys just keep adding to the list of things going wrong. The best preventative I know is a regular stretching routine. Start making it a habit to stretch out when you tune in.

Slow-Speed Topple

I crash quite a bit, but most of the time it's not with flames shooting out on screaming descents. It's on slow-speed technical sections. It's surprising how many collarbones have been broken by falls from a creeping roll or even a dead stop. The reason is the stiff, extended arm that transfers the impact to the shoulder. You lose your gyroscopic energy, lose your balance, fail to pull a foot off the pedal, and stick out an arm as you tip over. If it's not your collarbone that cracks, it may be your wrist.

Depending on what you're going to land on, one way to reduce the chance of serious damage is to hang on to the handlebar. Keep your hand on the grip and turn the bar so the end hits first. Ease yourself onto the ground by landing with your hip, arm, and shoulder in sort of a rolling motion. This technique works on soft surfaces, but you may need to use an outstretched arm if the ground is full of roots or rocks—things too hard for a hip to take. If you reach out, do your best to absorb the impact by collapsing your elbow, as if lowering yourself from a one-arm pushup.

Forward Dismount

A particularly bad crash is an endo on a downhill. You're usually going pretty fast, and there's an awful lot of air between where you launch and where you land. But if you keep your head, there's a very cool move that can prevent much pain and suffering.

What you can do is dismount over the front of the bike, land on your feet, and run down the hill till you regain control. It's one of those moves that you can't believe you just did. I've actually pulled it off a few times.

As the bike tips up on the front wheel, pull a foot and extend that leg over the handlebar. Take a giant step as the other foot releases, and leave the bike tumbling behind you. After that, you half-run, half-slide as you try

Tech Tip

What's the first thing you do during a crash? Besides scream, I mean. You put out your arms to break your fall. It's instinctive. And it can really cut up your hands if they aren't protected.

Cycling gloves come in various styles. I prefer the type with five full fingers or the type with a full thumb and four three-quarter-length fingers. Thumbs need full coverage for working the shifters without slipping or becoming raw or blistered.

Padding in the palm isn't necessary. In fact, it can be a drawback because it fills up your hands. The more material you're squeezing, the less feel you have on the grips and the more fatigue you develop in your forearms. Grips will provide all of the cushioning that your hands need if your front tire isn't overinflated and your suspension fork is properly tuned.

to stop. Whether you can actually stay on your feet depends on what the trail is throwing at you. Even if you fall, you won't be tangled up with the machinery, which is always good to avoid in crashes.

Remember this move the next time you find yourself in a downhill endo. Trying it is better than going over head first with the bike still attached.

Crash Course

Crashing and mountain biking may go hand in hand, but you can still do a lot to limit your time on the ground. Here's a collection of reminders.

Be honest about your abilities. Many a crash has occurred because a rider tried to do something that was beyond his skill level. When you get in over your head, your bike could soon be over your head, too.

Fatigue is another factor. When you can barely handle a risky section while fresh and strong, think twice about trying to ride it when your muscles are tired and your focus is fuzzy.

Take some risks. Healthy apprehension is one thing, but don't be afraid to take reasonable risks. This is how you learn and improve. You have to be willing to fall down once in awhile. Just do a smart job of picking your spots. You don't want to push the envelope beside a rocky ravine, but a sandy turn is quite forgiving. Go for it when it makes little difference if you mess up.

Get comfortable with wheel drift. Learn not to panic and grab the brakes in fast turns, or you'll suffer nasty consequences. Rely on a combination of countersteering and angulation to make it through.

Ride so the bike floats beneath you. Get into the attack position on choppy ground so you can soak up the chattering with bent arms and legs. Be ready to either jump over or suck up big bumps that could jeopardize your control.

Keep your cool in ruts. When the front wheel drops in, a common reaction is to immediately turn the handlebar sharply to get out. Boom—the wheel twists and over you go. Instead, stay in the rut until you can either stop and lift the bike out or until the walls taper enough for you to ride out.

Maintain clearance for your bar-ends. This applies for rides in the woods and other confined areas. If you snag a bar-end on a branch, the crash will be brutally sudden. Some of my most surprising wrecks have happened this way, including one at an off-road triathlon in Louisiana. After swimming a mile in a swamp, I'd been on the bike for about 90 minutes in very hot weather. I was getting sloppy on a trail that was unforgivingly tight through

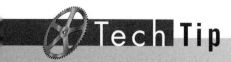

Tech Tip

Some equipment should be replaced routinely if you ride hard. You run the risk of brake failure, for instance, if you start a wet ride with brake pads that are already worn. Always buy replacement pads with a compound that matches the type of weather and soil that you ride in.

The chain is in danger of snapping if the links have been damaged by chainsuck. It will probably let go during a forceful pedal stroke, with potentially nasty results.

Because it can be catastrophic if a handlebar snaps, install a new one at least every two years (annually if you race). Be wary of lightweight replacement bars. The potential reduction in strength isn't worth the few grams of weight you'll save. Should you suffer a cartwheeling crash with heavy front-end impact, consider replacing the handlebar and even the fork right away.

Be skeptical about superlight equipment. I like titanium pedal axles for road riding, for instance, but I'm leery of their strength and durability for mountain biking unless I know that the engineers at Specialized have okayed them with a fatigue test. When thinking about lightweight parts, consider the manufacturer's reputation. Ask other riders about their experiences.

Finally, pay attention to the mechanical failures you see around you. When I pass a broken-down rider, I try to check the brand and model of the part that's involved. If I'm using the same part, I know to keep an eye on it. If I'm not, I may want to avoid it when I change equipment.

the trees. Next thing I knew, I was sliding through the pine needles on my shoulder. I didn't even have time to put out a hand. Bar-ends that curve inward are less apt to snag something than are the type that stick straight out.

Beware the brakes. Poor braking technique is a common cause of crashes. This is especially true for the front brake, which causes crashes when you use it too hard or in the wrong situations. I saw two guys have really bad crashes at the wicked Bailey's Bailout drop-off in Vail, Colorado. They grabbed too much front brake and cartwheeled a long way down.

Remember that sometimes the best way to regain control is to release the brakes so your wheels can roll. Control your speed in advance of technical sections where the wheels need to move freely for maneuverability.

Practice getting your feet out. Cleats are great for climbing power and descending control, but they also are a major reason that people crash, particularly when they're going so slowly that they lose their balance. The tendency in an emergency is to twist your feet out with upward force instead of keeping the rotation parallel to the pedals. The cleats don't release, and over you go. Develop the ability to instantly unclip either foot no matter what position it's in.

Be mindful of mud. It can hinder your ability to get out of the pedals even if you're using excellent technique. In the high desert of New Mexico, where I ride in winter, the soil is a combination of clay and sand. When it gets wet, it seems like epoxy between my shoes and pedals. Sometimes, I have to take my feet out of my shoes to separate myself from the bike. In evil mud conditions, try not to put yourself in situations that require instant release.

Take notice of pedal clearance. Sometimes, you need to coast or ratchet to keep your pedals from slamming into obstacles or banked turns. The timing is easier if you use a higher gear, because the pedals don't come around as quickly.

I often see guys bashing and crashing late in races. By then, their vision is blurred, their reactions are slower, and they're not paying attention to details. It's easy to pound a rock with a pedal or crankarm. The rear wheel lifts up, loses traction, and the bike pitches to the side. It happens so fast and unexpectedly that there's no chance to prevent a fall.

Space out. Whether you're racing or just riding with some friends, leave a margin for error between your front wheel and the bike just ahead. If the

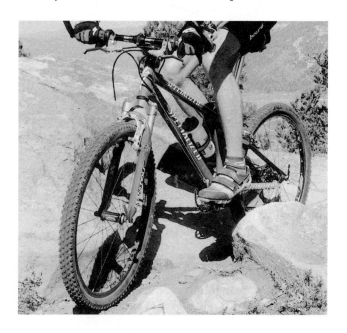

To prevent slamming a pedal into an obstacle, time your pedal stroke so it's up as you roll past, or ratchet the pedals back and forth with half-strokes.

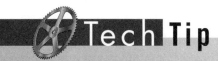

Tech Tip

Because mountain bikes suffer so much abuse, it's not uncommon for mechanical failures to cause crashes. Even though you're doing everything right as a rider, a part could break and put you down.

My philosophy is that you can never blame the bike. It's up to you to make sure that your equipment is in good condition and adjusted correctly. If you inspect your bike frequently and maintain it properly, equipment-related crashes should be very rare.

Pay special attention to your fork, handlebar, and stem. If one of these up-front parts fails, the crash can be catastrophic—you could go right onto your head. If you notice any strange noise or behavior, check it out immediately. I didn't one time, and it almost cost me dearly.

For several rides, I'd noticed creaking from my stem. It didn't seem important, so I let it go. Next, I found myself on a fast ride with friends on the Colorado Trail. We were smoking a tight, slightly downhill section when the creak suddenly became a metallic snap. "Hmmm," I thought, "That's a different sound." I came to the next turn but the bike wouldn't respond—it continued going straight. An internal stem bolt had broken. Turning the handlebar had no effect on the front wheel. Luckily, this section of trail was lined with scrub oak instead of the typical cliff exposure. I was able to ride it out and avoid a bad crash. Luck spared me a hospital visit, but I still had a long hike with a broken bike.

If you hear it, fear it. Then fix it before your next ride. Many times, a part will start making telltale noises before it lets go.

rider in front of you messes up and suddenly stops or goes down, you need a second to avoid a collision. The guy behind you should extend the same courtesy, so remind him, if necessary. It's nerve-wracking to feel like you'll be rear-ended if you bobble a move.

Come to think of it, I probably should have said something to my friend Martin Stenger near the top of a steep drop-off during a race in Durango, Colorado. He was hot on my wheel and rammed me when I slowed to set up for the chute. By the time my bike stopped cartwheeling down the hill, the chain was tied in a knot. I had to take it apart to fix it. I nicknamed Martin "PT-109" after that incident. Remember JFK's boat that was cut in half by a Japanese destroyer in World War II?

Beware of reckless riders. I ride with lots of people, but I avoid going with those who think that a ride isn't a real ride unless they draw blood. They seem bent on proving that they're not afraid of landing hard on sharp things. Personally, my idea of an enjoyable time is not pulling guys from the woods with broken legs or head injuries.

Wear body armor. If you're an aspiring downhiller, you're going to push the envelope and crash a lot in practice and events. To limit the damage, wear protective gear on your legs, arms, and torso. Use a full-face helmet, too. Besides reducing injuries, this will help you get accustomed to riding in exactly the same equipment that you race in.

Look where you want to go, not where you're afraid of going. I can't emphasize this enough. Violations of this rule probably cause more mistakes and crashes than any other reason. Concentrate on your line. Block out negative, fearful thoughts. I can assure you that this ability is shared by all the best riders.

Practice and then practice again. Ultimately, the best way to avoid crashing is to get good at every move in mountain biking. If you never crash, you aren't pushing yourself enough. There's a big difference, however, between taking calculated risks and crashing because your skills are underdeveloped.

19 Epic Rides

The Way to Make
Mountain Biking Last All Day

If there's one good thing about my racing career winding down, it's that I'll be able to enjoy more of those daylong, adventure-filled outings known as epic rides. I've always wanted to do more of them—after all, my Rocky Mountain backyard is full of opportunities. But as a guy who made his living by racing, I had to bag my enthusiasm. During the season, I couldn't risk the effects that too many six- or eight-hour rides would have on my legs. Cross-country races put a premium on speed and power, two aspects of performance that aren't helped by titanic cruises into the backcountry. Endurance, yes. Fresh, fast legs, no.

Epic rides are the equivalent of an endurance runner's long, steady distance workouts. They accustom your body to burning stored fat for fuel, sparing glycogen for the more intense efforts that push your heart rate past 65 percent of its max. After two to three hours of riding, your glycogen stores are nearly exhausted. And you will be, too, unless you efficiently metabolize body fat for energy and snack on foods and drinks rich in carbohydrates. This is the key to riding all day and feeling good doing it. The more rides over three hours you take, the more adept your body becomes at using fat for fuel. Simply put, you become a stronger, more efficient engine on your bike.

There's a psychological benefit, too. When you know that you can ride

Ned's KNOWLEDGE

If you're attracted to the adventure of epic rides, your first concern will probably be how to pedal for six hours if your average ride is two hours or less. For racers who want to improve endurance, the answer is easy: We hop on our road bikes and ramp up our mileage on pavement.

But what if you're a nonracing recreational mountain biker who doesn't own a road bike? In this case, your buildup to epic distances has to take place on your off-road machine. The key is to do one long ride each week, but not on terrain that will beat you up. If you don't care to ride on paved roads, use dirt roads. Rough and hilly trails aren't the right choice for this training, because they take too much out of you.

Increase the duration of your long ride by about 10 percent each week. This steady buildup will condition your mind, body, and metabolism to the special demands of an epic ride. Practice eating and drinking. Determine the foods that you digest well while riding.

Rule of thumb: Most people can handle a ride that's two to three hours longer than their average long training ride. So, once you build up to four hours, you should be ready for a fun and reasonably comfortable all-day outing—if you stay fueled, hydrated, and keep a sensible pace.

for four, five, or six hours without falling apart by the end, a two-hour ride or race becomes a lot less intimidating, even if you're going at a much faster pace. I also like the way that epic rides provide a different experience. You approach them thinking "distance" not "speed," which is kind of refreshing. And because long rides take you far from familiar trails, they put the adventure back into mountain biking.

Speaking of titanic cruises, you certainly want to avoid any sinking feelings on an epic ride. Despite all of the benefits, there are real risks. A desperate situation could result from such things as getting lost, running out of food or water, or suffering a bad injury or a mechanical breakdown. Preparation is key, and then it's a matter of smart riding.

Bike Check

A thorough preride bike inspection and correction usually will prevent major mechanical failures (with the exception of crashes). Remember that it's not just your own bike that you need to be concerned about—it's the bike of everyone who's riding with you. If one person has a major problem miles into the backcountry, it's your problem, too. You can't just ride off and leave him. His pace becomes your pace, so ride with people who maintain their equipment. Everyone must be as thorough with his preride check as when preparing for a race.

Pay close attention to your rear suspension, which has several moving parts that can loosen or wear out. Check for excessive play in the fork legs, which can cause seals to start leaking. Make sure the headset isn't loose, because looseness stresses the frame and fork. Look closely for cracks in the

TRUE STORY

A classic epic ride from my hometown of Durango in Colorado is called the Kennebec Pass loop. You head out of town and into La Plata Canyon before climbing to the top of the 13,000-foot pass. From there, you can get on the Colorado Trail. It's a spectacular ride with a ton of climbing. Depending on your pace, it will take you between 6 and 10 hours to get out and back.

Or it could take a couple of days. People get lost up there all the time. Several trails intersect, so it gets disorienting. The big mistake is turning away from Durango and dropping in on the wrong side of the divide. Once people realize their mistake, it takes a major effort to ride back up again. There's no way to get home before sundown.

One day, the search-and-rescue guys asked me to help them get two riders out. They wanted me to show them the area where people take the wrong trail. I drove part of the way up the pass, then got into a helicopter.

It was a superwindy day. At that altitude, the helicopter didn't have much power. We climbed toward a notch in the mountain, and everything seemed fine until we hit a downdraft. I could feel the chopper sinking. I could also see the pilot sweating. He fought with the stick as we jerked all over the sky. He couldn't turn around, because we would lose momentum and then really sink. We were so scared. I've never felt that helpless. Just as we were being pushed into the ridge, the downdraft eased and we made it over. When we finally landed, the co-pilot got out and immediately threw up.

Be responsible on epic rides. If you get lost or have a major problem far from the nearest help, you're not only putting your own safety at risk but you're also endangering everyone who tries to find you.

frame and fork. Find and fix any squeaks or creaks you've been hearing. See that all brake pads are contacting the rims squarely. Replace the pads if they're somewhat worn and the upcoming ride could be wet, muddy, or laced with long descents—conditions that eat pads fast. Go around the bike and put a wrench on every nut and bolt, checking for snugness. Inspect the tires for sidewall cuts and things stuck in the tread. Make sure the wheels are true and no spokes are loose or broken.

Equipment

I'm a big fan of using CO_2 cartridges to instantly inflate spare tubes in races. They're fine for epic rides, too. Using CO_2 may sound wasteful and expensive, but by paying close attention to the condition of my tires and using adequate pressure, I rarely get flats. In fact, the majority of my cartridges go to fellow riders whose pumps malfunction. Even if you use CO_2, at least one person should carry a pump. Flats could outnumber the cartridges that you pack. For the same reason, take a patch kit or two in addition to spare tubes. In case of a sidewall tear, carry some duct tape or other material that can be used to line the inside of a tire.

As for tools, don't go overboard. If the bikes check out okay before the ride, a standard tool kit with a selection of allen keys and a couple of screwdriver blades should be enough. Carry a chain tool and a spoke wrench, but unless you're going way out on a multi-day trip, I think it's overkill to pack spare cables, spokes, brake pads, and other parts.

A first-aid kit could come in handy, but it's hard to carry one in a jersey pocket or a seatbag. The best way to expand storage space is to wear a backpack-style hydration system that includes several pockets and chambers. You get greatly increased fluid-carrying capacity along with the room to take as much stuff as you can stand to have on your back. Include some iodine tablets in the first-aid kit in case you need to purify water.

If you're riding in an unfamiliar area—say, during a vacation—don't try a long ride without a map and compass. You're just begging to get lost without them. Check at the local bike or mountaineering stores for maps and advice on the best routes. A map that includes elevation lines will help you make smart decisions. The locals can also tip you off about areas to avoid (where the streams are too high, for instance) or trails where riding is prohibited.

A headlight that uses AA or C batteries is relatively small and lightweight. Its burn time (at least three hours for most models) is good insurance on a ride that will push the limits of daylight. To save space in your pockets, carry the light in its handlebar bracket.

Cellular phones are becoming common in the backcountry. I've seen them used by equestrians and hunters. They're easy to carry, but they aren't always effective in the mountains. You may have to walk or ride to the top of a ridge to get a connection, like pro racer Travis Brown's father had to do. He fell into a ravine while hiking in a remote area, breaking his leg and twisting his back. He had a cellular phone but couldn't get reception. By crawling a couple of hundred feet up the hillside, he was able to contact help and save his life.

Carry some waterproof matches. If you need to spend the night, a fire is a nice luxury. During the day, the smoke curling up can help rescuers find you if you're hurt and unable to get out by yourself.

Clothing

Avoid wearing something brand-new, particularly untried shorts or shoes, on a long ride. A seam or pressure in the wrong place can become more than an annoyance as the day wears on.

Be sure your shoes are comfortable for walking. Some models are pretty narrow in the toebox, which is fine for riding but not for hiking. The tread should provide good traction, because you'll need it in places that force you off the bike. Select a jersey made of material that wicks moisture. It'll keep you more comfortable than simple spandex will. Also, make sure the jersey has relatively roomy pockets for carrying food and spare clothes. I long ago stopped buying jerseys with small or tight pockets.

Check the weather report to learn if any changes are expected. A lot can happen in six to eight hours. A weather front moving through can turn a sunny morning into a windy, rainy afternoon with plunging temperatures. Hypothermia, a condition in which the body's core temperature plummets to life-threatening levels, can occur quickly. It's a major danger to those of us who ride in the Rockies.

Even if no risky weather is expected, pack a rain jacket. This is my biggest concession to riding into the backcountry. I make sure the material is actually waterproof, not just water resistant. It may be a bit hot for riding, but its protection could be vital if I wind up spending the night out there. Nonporous material will retain body heat.

On a day when there could be a wide swing in temperatures, use arm and leg warmers. They're effective at keeping the chill off, and they roll up small enough to fit in a jersey pocket when you don't need them. Likewise, consider taking regular gloves and a polypropylene hat or balaclava that fits under your helmet. If your fingers go numb from the cold, you can't shift or brake properly. You can lose lots of body heat through your head, especially in the rushing air of a long descent if you're wet from sweat or rain. Even a thin polypro cap will make a big difference, and it's easy to store.

Food and Drink

You'll be burning around 500 calories per hour on an all-day ride. You need to replace the majority of them so your energy level stays high. Bonking in the woods with the sun setting and two hours left to ride is no way to end the day.

Load your muscles with glycogen, their favorite fuel, by eating heartily during the two to three days before the ride. Emphasize foods that are rich in carbohydrates—pasta, cereals, bread, potatoes, fruits—and don't skip dessert. Drink plenty of water and beverages without caffeine or alcohol to ensure that you're fully hydrated.

On the morning of an epic ride, enjoy an epic breakfast. You won't be sprinting from a starting line. It's okay if you begin the ride with a fairly full stomach. Eat foods that you know will agree with you, and consider the advice of my friend Skip Hamilton. Skip is a coach and incredible masters athlete who has many victories in running, cycling, and cross-country skiing. High among his laurels are four victories in the 100-mile foot race at 10,000-foot Leadville, Colorado. To fuel such efforts, Skip is a big believer in complementing his pre-event high-carbo meals with protein and some fat. For instance, he'll add an omelet to his prerace pancakes. The benefit, he says, is "compact calories and a longer burn."

Try it and see. It works for me, Ed Pavelka, and other riders we know. My stomach can feel hollow only two hours after an all-pancake breakfast, but add the eggs, cheese, and maybe some yogurt, and I'm good all morning.

During a long ride, I prefer solid food instead of energy gel, my usual race diet. "Chew food" just sticks with me longer. I like dried fruit, and energy bars work well because they're easy to carry and they pack lots of calories for their size. In addition, bars give you a wide choice of nutrients. Depending on what your experience proves best, you can eat a bar that's virtually all carbohydrates or one that has a relatively high percentage of protein. Some bars even give you a hefty dose of fat, creating a longer energy release.

I never take plain water on a long ride. Instead, I use a sports drink. Why drink something with no calories when you can simultaneously stay hydrated and get about 150 calories per bottle? Unless you carry a water filter or are certain to encounter a campground or other source of potable water, you need to be a two-wheeled tank truck. Besides filling your two bike-mounted bottles, wear a hydration pack. Most of them hold 70 to 100 ounces. Even this much may not be enough during summer temperatures at high altitude. Don't risk running out. In addition to the riding and off-bike time you expect, factor in the crash or mechanical problem that could keep you in the woods even longer.

Within an hour after the ride, get a good amount of carbohydrates back into your system. Your muscles are depleted of glycogen at this point,

Ned's KNOWLEDGE

A new type of competition has been snowballing in popularity—ultradistance races. These are like epic rides for prizes. There are two main forms: solo races such as the Leadville 100 (miles) in Colorado, and 24-hour races for relay teams. In 1999, there were 10 such events nationwide.

The solo races should be approached much like any long ride. It's pacing rather than pure speed that determines how well you do. Much of the general advice for epic rides applies. Bike preparation and caloric intake are very important. One advantage in a race is the availability of food and water at checkpoints along the course. You should carry some emergency food, but you don't need to pack a full-day's supply.

Some 24-hour relay races attract thousands of competitors. Typically, there are four people on a team, each taking turns on a loop that takes about an hour to ride. Once you finish a lap, you have three hours to recover, rehydrate, and refuel. In addition to the fitness it takes to ride hard for an hour, you need the stamina to do it six times, around the clock. Also essential is a reliable lighting system that's bright enough to let you go as fast as you can without danger.

Team races are great fun because you share the experience with friends. The start/finish area is often like a cross between a rock-music festival and a campground, with so many tents, vans, and people. Solo races, on the other hand, emphasize individual qualities. Not many riders can actually contend for first place in a race that takes so long. Instead, you win by meeting your time goal or, as in any epic ride, by simply reaching the finish line.

making them very receptive to being refueled. By taking advantage of this period, known as the glycogen window, you will recover quicker and have some life in your legs the next day. I like to down a bottle of a high-carbo sports drink right after finishing, then have a high-carbo meal after cleaning up. This meal also includes a good source of protein to help repair any muscle damage.

The meal is the next-to-last step in recovering from a long ride or race. The final step is the one you don't actually take: Try to stay off your feet for the rest of the day. You can do this on a stool at the local tavern if you like, assuming you're not in serious training. Hoisting a couple of cold ones with your pals is one way to celebrate an epic ride.

Pace

A long ride and a race are similar in one respect. As each goes on, you need to continually assess how you're holding up. Don't kid yourself. Don't tell yourself, "I'm fine. I don't have to stop. I can push a little farther." You need to make realistic evaluations of how your legs are doing. Are they tired or tight? How's your food and fluid intake? If you let yourself become fatigued and depleted to the point of cramping, it's going to be very hard to continue.

Good pacing on a long ride means stopping occasionally to rest, stretch, and refuel. Let beautiful spots like overlooks or waterfalls remind you to relax and enjoy the scenery. Good pacing also means never pushing your effort to the point at which you go anaerobic. This level of exertion is fueled solely by glycogen and quickly burns your precious reserves. The biggest risk occurs on climbs. Keep your heart rate below the 80 to 85 percent of max that causes your anaerobic energy system to fire up. If you start panting and your legs are burning, immediately back off. Remember, you're not in a race. You're a winner on this day if you finish with a grin and a little energy to spare.

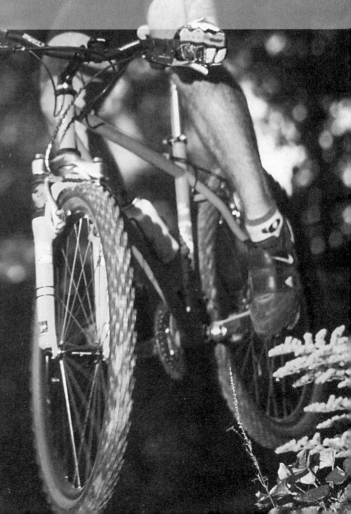

Part Three

Competition

20 Racing Opportunities

Winning Is Just One of Many Reasons to Compete

Should you race? It's not for everyone, so I don't want to push you into it. But at the same time, I can tell you that it will enrich you with cycling experiences that you can't get any other way.

Let me give you an example. At the Grundig World Cup in Mont Ste. Anne, Quebec, I got strapped into a roller-coaster ride of emotions that I'll never forget. Soon after the start, it began pouring rain—the heaviest I've ever ridden in. A sheet of water was pouring from the front of my helmet. It was so bad that I was laughing.

Pretty soon, Jan Wiejak passed me. My nickname for him is Weedwhacker. We exchanged places eight or nine times, trying to get rid of each other. If I slid out on a slimy root, he jumped off his bike and ran past me. We banged handlebars sliding down the treacherous hills. But we were enjoying it. I'd say, "Not you again, Weedwhacker." We actually worked our way up to fifth or sixth position.

But with a lap to go, we both blew at the same time. As the other riders passed, we stopped worrying about each other and concentrated on surviving. We walked sections of the course that we had ridden earlier. But we finished. And at the end, we patted each other on the back. We respected the experience we'd just shared. Neither of us was satisfied with his result, but enduring to the end was a victory in itself. That's racing—the best and the worst of it.

153

Reasons to Race

Road racing is tough to get into, because it requires very specialized skills. The dangers and tactics of wheel-to-wheel pack riding intimidate almost every newcomer. But mountain bike racing is different. Unlike road racing, it's tactically simple and emphasizes your personal ability, not group dynamics. After the big starting bunch thins out, it's primarily you versus the course. Because drafting rarely offers a significant advantage and the riders are usually spread out, one guy's screwup doesn't mean a big crash for the people behind him. This also results in less antagonism and more camaraderie.

Racing pushes the envelope of your bike-handling skills. Some guys may be able to whip you on the local downhills when you're out cruising, but many things change when your heart rate is 185 beats per minute for an hour. Bike control is one of them. You develop a special skill by negotiating trails while you're fatigued and in oxygen debt.

Racing takes you to a new fitness level. Many riders will never discover their maximum cardiovascular potential until they race. It usually won't happen in training, because reaching heart rates that high takes too much intentional suffering. Racing finds your redline automatically.

You won't know how good you really are until someone who is better pushes you. I'd been racing mountain bikes for three years when John Tomac came on the scene. Here was a kid with great climbing prowess and incredible descending ability. He basically said, "You guys have to step up to a new level. You can't win anymore if you're just a climber." I became a better all-around racer because of John.

You'll learn a lot more about equipment. As a former motorcycle mechanic, I love the challenge of suspension setup, tire selection, and drivetrain choice. There's a lot you can do to customize your bike to perform better on a given course. There's gratification in that. Like me, you may become a rider who finds nearly as much enjoyment in tinkering with a bike as in riding it.

If you like traveling, racing is your ticket to some of the most scenic areas of the country. You'll get to experience the best of Colorado, Utah, California, Vermont, West Virginia—places with sensational singletrack and classic events. You'll be exposed to vastly different terrain, which will help you develop more complete bike-handling skills. Even in your own region, races will introduce you to great trails that you may not otherwise find out about. You can go back anytime for recreational rides.

Ned's KNOWLEDGE

Whether you race or not, it's hard to put enough emphasis on the benefits of traveling to other regions of the country. If you always ride where you live, you'll be missing out on so much. Around my hometown in Colorado, for example, the trails are high, dry, and rocky. When I go to Vermont to race, the air is thick with humidity and the singletrack is wet, slippery, and criss-crossed with roots. It's a challenge to be able to go fast in both places. I get real satisfaction from adapting to the differences in bike setup and riding techniques.

If you live east, go west. If you live north, go south. This is what I call destination mountain biking. It makes our sport an adventure, whether you're traveling to compete or to spend a week of vacation. Besides the terrain change, you encounter different people, attitudes, and customs. It's an education you can't get except by being there.

As I look back over my racing career, it's astonishing how many trips I've taken around the country and the world. The experiences have enriched my life in ways that I could never have imagined. I encourage you to travel with your bike, too, as much as you can.

Finally, there's the satisfaction of passing a tough test. Take it from me, there's nothing like the feeling of accomplishment that you have as you finish the last lap of a difficult race.

Attitude Is Everything

To make racing a fun experience that turns you into a better rider, remember these points.

Be patient. Your early races should be considered tests against the field of riders and the course. Consider how many riders you beat, not just how many beat you. Remember, poor performances can be the best learning experiences.

Finish each race. Otherwise, you shouldn't bother to go through all the preparation, travel, and expense. Lots of riders quit because they get too far behind the leaders or because the people whom they think they should be beating are ahead of them. So what? Keep riding. Even if I bonk and have to lie down beside the trail, I get up and finish.

Leave the excuses behind. There are three words that you hear from some people after every race: coulda, woulda, shoulda. In order to make racing a positive experience, you have to take the blame for everything that goes wrong. It doesn't matter if a shop worked on your bike, it's still your responsibility. The same goes for crashing. Some riders treat crashes as if they have nothing to do with them, blaming their bikes or other riders. Remember, wrecks happen. You can avoid most of them by riding smart and with finesse.

Reflect on your performance. Sit back and look at your race as if through someone else's eyes. Did you lose time on the descents? Did you fail to keep momentum in switchbacks? Take time to examine every as-

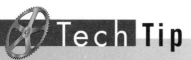

You don't need the latest and greatest bike to start racing. You'll see more benefits from developing skills and fitness than from investing big bucks in fancy equipment. It's the motor that counts the most.

However, if your bike isn't light enough (under 26 pounds) or reliable enough for competition, you should upgrade to a model in the midprice range, say $900 to $1,200. You could spend a lot less or a lot more, but in this range, you get durability and performance that should let you get the most out of your developing skill. In other words, the bike won't hold you back. Beginners don't really need to spend more, because as bike prices increase, refinements become less noticeable. The pros seek every little edge, and their bikes can cost up to $4,000. As you move beyond $1,500 or so, the improvements aren't cost-effective for recreational racers.

Although the trend is inexorably toward dual suspension, I'm not ready just yet to condemn hardtails for racing. In general, a bike with only front suspension is lighter than one with dual suspension, and it gives you a fast, efficient ride in terrain that's not overly rough. Race courses, though, tend to be the most jagged terrain that promoters can find. For this reason, a dualie may be the best bike if you will be traveling to compete.

Remember the two big advantages to dual suspension. First, you can stay seated on rough surfaces and thus conserve energy that you would burn by standing. Second, you can descend faster as the rear wheel follows the contour of the ground and insulates your legs from the pounding. The main disadvantage occurs if the rear suspension moves a lot during pedaling, especially during out-of-saddle climbing. This energy-sapping problem can result from poor design, improper adjustment, or both.

If you're staying local, test-ride both types of bikes, check with area racers to

pect. Make notes so you can review these lessons even after time has blurred the specifics. Careful reflection can turn mistakes into positive learning experiences.

Race for the right reasons. You shouldn't compete if you really don't want to. Don't let peer pressure or machismo drive you to the starting line. It has to be your decision. I've always loved the challenge of seeing how fit I can become, and racing is the best way to reach my potential. I know that this reason isn't enough for everyone. If you try racing and decide you don't like it, that's good enough for me. You gave it a shot, so you have my respect.

see what they ride, and read reviews in the bike magazines. Different rear-suspension designs usually have different performance characteristics. One brand of dualie may work much better with your riding style and terrain than another brand.

If you decide to go with a hardtail, you can still get some dualie benefits with a shock-absorbing seatpost. There are two types: one telescopes in line with the seat tube, moving vertically, and the other pivots rearward on a parallelogram linkage. I like the latter because it moves horizontally to accommodate the force that your butt puts on the saddle when you hit a bump. It doesn't alter seat height nearly as much as the telescoping type does. Whichever design you choose, make sure it provides damping to prevent kickback after compression.

If you stick with your present bike, you may be able to boost its performance with some intelligent weight reduction. A lighter bike climbs better, of course, but there's more to it than that. Concentrate on the parts that rotate. The lighter they are, the less energy it takes to keep them turning. That's why wheels are key. You can buy racing wheels with lightweight rims and spokes; or you can improve your present wheels by installing lighter tires and tubes. By the way, hub weight isn't much of a concern, because it's at the center of the wheel. It barely contributes to the weight that you must rotate.

Lighter pedals and shoes reduce the energy it takes to turn the crankarms. The rule of thumb is to spend your upgrade money on rotating parts before buying something static like a superlight seatpost or handlebar. You also need to consider the durability of any weight-saving item. Even though upgrade parts are usually expensive, they may break more easily or wear out sooner because they're so light. If you have a limited amount of money, you don't want to have to replace your replacement parts.

License to Thrill

About 30,000 mountain bikers belong to NORBA (National Off-Road Bicycling Association), the governing body of U.S. off-road racing. To compete in a NORBA race (there are more than a thousand each year), you need to purchase a license. The cost as of late 1998 was $30 per year. If you're not quite ready to take the plunge, you can buy a one-day trial license at any race site.

One great thing about NORBA's setup is the variety of classes and categories. No matter what your age, sex, or skill level, you won't be thrown in with a bunch of people of completely different abilities and experience. Racing classes are termed junior (age 18 and under), senior (19 to 34), veteran (35 to 44), and master (45 and over). These classes are further divided into five categories: beginner (first-timers and local recreational racers), sport (intermediate regional racers), expert (advanced regional and national racers), semi-pro (aspiring pros), and pro (the best national and international racers). In addition to the classic cross-country race on a lap course, NORBA's event lineup includes the point-to-point race, hill climb, downhill, dual slalom, stage race, ultra-endurance race (more than 75 miles), 24-hour relay, and observed trials. When you join NORBA, you receive a monthly publication that lists all the races around the country and keeps you up-to-date on the news of the sport.

Is this fun or what? Racing will give you mountain biking experiences (as well as a level of fitness) that you can't get any other way.

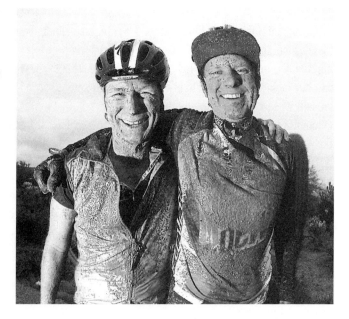

The beginner class is exactly what it sounds like. To make sure that improving riders don't dwell in beginner and hog all the top prizes, a rider must advance to the sport category after placing in the top five in five beginner races. On the other hand, if you feel that you're good enough, you can start racing in the expert category right away. The catch is that you can't downgrade to sport or beginner if you discover that this was a mistake. My advice is to start at beginner and work your way up. If you're good enough to race in expert, you'll be there soon enough.

You should also become involved in your local off-road cycling scene. Check at a bike shop to find out about mountain bike–club activities. There may be weekly training sessions or practice races. Club-level racing is low-pressure, and it's affordable because there's no travel or pricey entry fees. Hanging with experienced racers is the quickest way to learn the ins and outs of the sport. This applies not only to techniques and strategy but also to tips on equipment, tires, suspension setup, and other mechanical aspects that help improve your performance but are hard to figure out on your own.

To learn more about the structure and rules of mountain bike racing or to request a NORBA license application, write to the USA Cycling License Desk, One Olympic Plaza, Colorado Springs, CO 80909. Information about NORBA is available on the Web at www.usacycling.org/mtb/. Also, check at local bike shops and clubs. Some are NORBA members and have literature and license forms on hand.

21 Race-Day Tactics

Start Fast and Finish Strong in Cross-Country Races

Thirty seconds before the gun at a World Cup race in Mammoth, California, my heart rate rose from the adrenaline as I ran down a mental checklist: I'd memorized the course, warmed up, selected the right start gear, and lined up on the outside to avoid midpack pileups.

The gun went off. The rubber cord stretching across the front line released. I clipped in and started to sprint, then I watched in disbelief as the cord rebounded and got tangled in my wheel. By the time I dismounted and pulled out the cord, 130 guys had a 15-second head start—a racer's nightmare and a great example of how even when you've prepared perfectly, the unthinkable can happen.

Fortunately, two of my teammates—talented downhill specialists Todd Tanner and the late Jason McRoy—were racing the cross-country just to get workouts. I tucked in behind them, took some very unorthodox lines, and by the time we hit the climbs, we'd passed more than half of the field. I finished in eighth place (second American), and a disastrous start turned into some valuable World Cup points.

Mountain bike racing is always a wild time. You never know the next thing that's going to be under your wheels (or in your spokes). Endless challenges are created by the course, your unique strengths and weaknesses, and the actions of riders around you. Whether you're a beginner, sport, or expert racer, here are my best tips for improving your chances.

Tapering

You should think of an important race as starting 7 to 10 days earlier than the scheduled date. This is when you need to adjust your training so you arrive at the line feeling strong and fresh. This process is called tapering—reducing the volume and intensity of training.

The right amount of tapering varies among individuals. It depends on how you're accustomed to training as well as on your physical condition going into race week. The trick is to taper enough to feel refreshed but not so much that you end up feeling lethargic.

My technique is to reduce the duration of training rides but continue making hard efforts. As the week progresses, I ride shorter distances while including some intervals or climbing to keep my lungs open and blood flowing. These short anaerobic periods prevent sluggishness and sharpen fitness. You have to be careful, though. This exertion must not come close to exhausting you. It's easy to get carried away and go too hard late in the week because you're feeling so good. Don't let your best performance happen on a training ride. Hold back and stay hungry for the real thing.

If you want a day off, take it two days before the race. If you don't ride the day before, your body may feel stale when the gun sounds. I like to take a short ride on the course on the eve of a race. After an easy warmup, I do a couple of one-minute all-out efforts. This opens me up and reminds my body of what it feels like to go hard. Then I ride easy for 15 to 20 minutes to relax and cool down.

If you compete frequently, it's not a good idea to taper fully for every race. The long-term result may very well be loss of strength and fitness. You need full training weeks to keep improving. Do some races for experience and a good hard workout. Train right through them by doing short two- or three-day tapers that return some snap to your legs and keep you from overtraining. Save full tapers for special events.

Fueling

Eat meals high in carbohydrates for several days before the race. Nothing extreme is necessary, just make sure to include foods such as pasta, rice, potatoes, cereals, bread, vegetables, and fruits. And don't forget some dessert. If you're tapering for an event, you burn fewer calories, so you may want to decrease meal portions slightly. You don't want to feel heavy as the race approaches.

My favorite meal on the eve of a race centers around pasta. There's no need to eat a big meal the next morning. In fact, it can be counterproductive. An early start time won't allow for complete digestion (and neither will a nervous stomach). You certainly don't want to taste breakfast again during the sprint from the starting line. Eat a light meal of easily digestible foods—the ones that experience has proven agree with you—at least two hours before the race. Three hours is safer. Good choices include fruit, oatmeal, yogurt, and bagels.

Always start a race well-hydrated. Take in plenty of fluids during the preceding two days. I like to get some extra calories and nutrients by using sports drinks, not just water. It's hard to actually overhydrate, but I once proved that it can be done. At a race in Mount Snow, Vermont, we expected record heat and humidity, so I drank and drank in the hours before the start. On the first hill, I was so bloated that I couldn't breathe. My stomach wasn't able to absorb all the water that I'd poured in. After the race, officials were taking dehydrated riders to the medical tent for intravenous fluids, but I was still sloshing. It's kind of funny now, but it was one of the worst finishes of my career.

On race day, stop your fluid intake about 30 minutes before the start, then drain off the excess shortly before you go to the line. Start sipping again while you're lined up, then drink wherever the course gives you a chance. During the inspection laps before a race, it's smart to identify smoother, flatter sections as reminders to take a swallow. Plenty of guys forget all about drinking until they feel thirsty late in the race. By then, they're dehydrated and their performance is suffering.

Inspecting

A typical course inspection involves riding a few laps with your buddies on the day before the race, following the most obvious lines. But doing it right means completing at least one lap alone so you can focus on the track. Things to think about include passing lanes, places where you'll need to shift to the small chainring, smooth spots for braking traction, easy sections where you can drink, and the best lines for maximizing momentum. Also think about how the course may change after hundreds of tires have rolled over it.

Make a note of the areas that lead into singletrack so you can surge around other riders and not get bogged down behind them. In the tight sections, look for places where the trail widens a bit or where there is firm ground beside it. If you know these spots beforehand, you can pick the right gear and build speed for a pass.

If the race is on Sunday, I like to arrive early enough on Friday to do my scouting laps. I don't have to worry much about using energy, because I still have Saturday to recover. On Saturday, I usually do one lap to keep my body open and confirm my lines. I continue looking for visual cues on or beside the trail to remind me of the gear that I need to shift to or the technique that I need to use.

During your scouting laps, you may recognize a better line that no one is using. It's a departure but it's still within the ribbons that define the course. Check it out visually, maybe even walk it, but don't ride it. Save it for race day. If you practice this line, other riders will see your wheel tracks and follow them. Your advantage will be lost.

Warming Up

A cross-country race is a time trial that starts with a field sprint. Although you'll eventually need to pace yourself for the distance and terrain, your start must be fast to get ahead of the inevitable bottleneck where singletrack begins. This makes it important to warm up well and then get to the starting area in time for a place in or near the front line.

I like to warm up for 40 minutes, including 25 minutes of easy riding and a couple of gradually increasing efforts of 1 to 2 minutes. I want to take my heart rate to about 85 percent of maximum. Then I ride easy for about 10 minutes to cool down. This prevents my legs from tightening too much while I wait for the gun. In chilly weather, I wear extra clothing until there's only a couple of minutes to go, then I hand it to a friend.

Starting

The front row is best, but only a fraction of the field will fit there. I like to line up near the front but toward the side. If other racers lock handlebars and pile up in front of me, it's easier to go around the outside. If the course quickly turns to the left, line up on the right so you can go around congestion in the apex, and vice versa. It helps to watch other classes of racers start, and learn from what you see.

If you can't get on the course to experiment with starting gears, find a spot with a similar slope. A low gear may be good for the first 10 yards, but then you'll lose ground when you shift. A low gear may also make it difficult to locate your pedal and clip in, because you won't be exerting much downward pressure. Conversely, a gear that's too high will prevent fast acceleration. By the time you get up to speed, many people will have ridden around you.

Practice 50-yard drag races with your friends to find the gears and techniques that work best for starting. To make it easier to clip in, set the pedal so it comes around horizontal on the push-off stroke. Let's say you start with your left foot clipped in and just past the top of the pedal circle, ready to exert a downstroke to get you moving. When the right pedal comes up, you want it to be flat or tilted slightly backward, not on edge. This helps your shoe's cleat find the pedal to clip in. If your cleat doesn't engage instantly, don't panic or pause to look down. Keep your head up to see the action around you, and keep pedaling to gain momentum while wiggling your foot until the cleat snaps in.

I like to sprint out of the saddle for about the first 50 yards. Using my whole body this way helps me generate speed. Other guys prefer to sit. Try it both ways to see which suits you. Either way, shift progressively to higher gears to maximize speed and prevent spinning out.

As important as technique is judging how hard to exert yourself. The start always requires speed, but let's say the course is fairly open for a mile or so before it narrows down. You can afford to leave the line a bit slower to avoid going anaerobic, then pick it up. Quite a few guys may pass you, but as you pace yourself, they'll bury themselves. You'll get some of them back

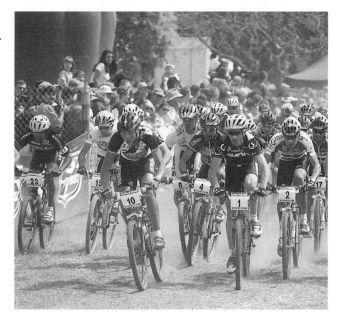

The start of a cross-country race is chaotic. But just like Tinker Juarez staying out of trouble, at far left, there's a lot you can do to emerge from the stampede in good position for a great performance.

TRUE STORY

The start of a race is emotionally charged. The first few seconds can make or break your chance for a good result, especially when something crazy happens.

Case in point: the 1991 NORBA point series final at Colorado's Purgatory ski area. I was going for my fifth national championship, but it wouldn't be easy. Several other guys were in strong contention. One was Daryl Price, a top pro for many years and my teammate at that time. On that course, it was important to get off the line fast because the starting area quickly angled in from both sides to start the singletrack.

There were about 25 of us packed tightly in the front row when the gun fired. One guy, a notoriously fast starter, was lined up toward the side. He barely had a lead when he veered across the pack toward the singletrack opening. He basically chopped the entire field. Daryl crashed in front of me and I slammed his butt with my front wheel. What a pileup. His rear derailleur was tangled in my spokes, so we couldn't quickly pull the bikes apart. Meanwhile, most of the field was disappearing.

To make matters worse, Daryl, normally a mild-mannered guy, lost control. He was hopping around and screaming unprintable things at the rider who caused this mess. It was a classic case of being frustrated, getting mad, and losing focus.

Blowing up in the heat of the moment is understandable, but never excusable. You simply can't let it happen. All you're doing is hurting yourself. Focus on your performance, no matter what. Daryl, who was only 19 at the time, did learn self-control. This race became a valuable lesson—and that's why he was such a good rider for so long.

Instead of losing my cool and making the damage worse by jerking the bikes apart, I used my experience from a few other rotten starts. First, I calmed Daryl down so we could get going again. I resisted the temptation to chase all-out. More than two hours of racing remained. I'd ridden the course, so I knew there were good places to pass. It looked bad with a hundred guys in front of me, but by the end, I'd picked off every one of them. Not far behind was Daryl, in fifth place.

before the singletrack starts, then pick off more from there to the finish. I've seen this strategy work many times. Remember, everyone has a finite amount of energy. By holding back early, you have more left during the latter part of the race when the dragsters are out of gas.

I'm not a very fast starter. I'm a come-from-behind rider who is rarely in the lead of any race at the halfway point. I get to the front either by coming on strong later in the race or by staying steady and catching fast starters who fade. If a course has few good places to pass, however, this isn't the best strategy. I may get trapped while the leaders are free to ride at speed. In this case, the solution is to put more effort into the start to get ahead of more people right away.

Look for a good wheel to draft if the speed is high and it's a long way to the singletrack. As on the road, drafting lets you ride with about 20 percent less effort than the guy in front. Just make sure he's a strong and confident rider. If he begins to blow or acquiesce to other riders, he'll take you back with him. Should you sense this happening, get around him right away and latch on to a different locomotive.

If your start isn't good and you find yourself near the back of a big field, forget about drafting. Instead, move toward the side where you have the clearest path for passing. This also will keep you out of the pileups that happen when someone's screwup causes a chain reaction through the pack.

Be aggressive about holding the position you want. If you back off when a guy comes up beside you, you'll be at the rear of the field in no time. Keep your speed and let people know that you're not going anywhere but forward. Attitude counts for a lot. Make people work hard to get past you.

Shifting

Anyplace where you have to shift to the small chainring is a potential trouble spot. Chainsuck is the main risk. It could force you to stop to unjam the chain—or worse, it could result in damage that causes shifting problems or even knocks you out of the race. Another danger with this shift is dropping the chain down around the bottom bracket. You have to stop and put it back on by hand.

Avoid these risks and maximize your momentum by staying in your middle and large chainrings as much as possible. If you need to go to the small chainring, don't wait so late to shift that you can't take pressure off the pedals. When you're pushing hard on a climb, the chain is under so much tension that the front derailleur can't drop it off the middle ring, keeping you in a gear that's too big. On short downhills, shift to a bigger gear even if only for a few pedal revolutions. This saves energy by building momentum that carries you farther up the next climb.

For racing, I use an 11-32 or 12-32 cogset with a 22T small chainring, 32T middle ring, and 44T big ring. This produces a 22x32T granny gear that I never use, not even on the steepest climbs, but it provides a 32x32T one-to-one ratio off my middle ring. This is low enough to let me ride up most hills without a risky shift onto the small chainring.

Don't be reluctant to use the big-chainring/big-cog crossover gear for brief periods. It's handy in races because it keeps you on the big chainring more and reduces the number of front shifts. Just be sure that your chain is long enough to shift in and out of the big/big combo without jamming.

Pacing

Those muffled explosions heard around any race course are the sound of riders blowing up. They're sort of a combination of a wheeze, a sigh, and a moan. Energy is gone, and the race changes to a test of survival. I know because it's happened to me more times than I like to remember.

To prevent this meltdown, it helps to be well-trained and well-rested before the race. Even if you're in top shape, though, you can still blow up if you don't pace yourself. The goal is to apportion your energy in a way that lets you go hard to the end and finish with your needle just touching on empty.

The ability to do this comes from experience—training and racing enough to know the limits of your strength and endurance. You need discipline to resist the early excitement that can sucker you into starting too fast. You need the awareness to back off whenever you're riding dangerously close to your redline.

A heart-rate monitor is one way of knowing but, because it's risky to look down at it during a race, an even better indicator is how hard you're breathing and how your legs feel. A burning tightness from lactic acid accumulation in your muscles is a sure sign that you're burying yourself.

The pace of most races goes like this: The first lap is the fastest because of the frenzied start and surging adrenaline. The second lap settles down as racers figure out their paces and pull back a bit to devise their strategies. The last lap can produce lots of shuffling as fast starters fade and riders who've paced themselves come on strong. If the race is one big loop instead of laps, expect it to break into thirds along the same lines.

As the race wears on, keep shifting in order to stay in gears that let you pedal efficiently. It's better to use gears that are a bit too low rather than too high, at least until you reach the point where you can go for broke to the finish. If you adapt yourself to this pedaling style in training, spinning lower gears conserves energy without necessarily hurting your speed.

Use the terrain to your advantage. It's more energy-efficient to make time on gradual climbs, descents, and flats, rather than on steep climbs.

This is why I have a reputation for spinning on tough hills. If you want to catch or leave a guy, it takes a lot more energy to increase speed on a hard climb than on milder parts of the course. My strategy is to ride steadily up tough hills but not slowly enough to lose time. I push over the tops and really work my gears on less vertical sections. Meanwhile, other guys push on steep climbs, then rest over the tops and in places where I'm honking on it. Lots of successful attacks are made at the tops of hills where riders who pushed too hard have no energy left to respond.

Resting

To race well, you need to identify spots on the course where you can recover slightly. I also create opportunities by easing into hard hills before spinning up them. You never want to be buried when you start a long climb.

Many riders expend more energy than necessary, especially on climbs and downhills. These sections create energy-sapping tension for different reasons. On climbs, riders tend to grimace. Jaws clench and neck veins bulge. The tension travels up from rigid arms into shoulders and chests, and lungs can't fully expand. The overall result is restricted breathing. Stay aware of this natural tendency to lock up. Fight it by concentrating on deep breathing, which can't be done with a tense jaw and chest. I use the simple yoga technique of consciously relaxing my upper body with a forced exhalation. This little trick also helps me drift off to sleep when I'm all wound up the night before a race.

On downhills, riders can seize up from anxiety or just plain fear, turning the descent into one long isometric contraction. This greatly reduces recovery from the climbing effort. They reach the bottom with nearly the same high heart rates that they had at the top. Obviously, you need to control your bike and continue to pedal, but you can also recover if you're relaxed and fluid. If you have difficulty descending this way in a race, devote more training time to the skills discussed in chapter 14.

Dismounting

If there's a hard climb that you can't ride more than half the time in practice, it will probably be faster to dismount and run up the hill in the race. Save time by jumping off before it gets too steep, rather than waiting until you're at a standstill and all momentum is gone. Think of the situation you're in when this happens. The bike wants to rear up in front and roll back down the hill. You have to get a foot out, then swing a leg over. It's tough to do this while a bike is trying to reverse its direction. Anticipate dismounts and make them during the run-in to vertical sections, where they're less awkward. Ultimately, you save time.

To dismount correctly, don't shift all the way down to your granny gear before you get off. This way, you're in a better ratio for starting up on the flat top or descent. Otherwise, you waste time by spinning.

To dismount on a climb, squeeze both brakes to prevent the bike from rolling back. Lean forward to keep the front end on the ground. Step off to the high side of the trail or away from any object that could cause a problem. Swing your other leg over, release the brakes, and hustle to a spot where you can hop on and start riding again. Push the bike with both of your hands on the grips or with one hand on the nearest grip and the other behind the saddle.

Practice dismounting to each side so you're adept no matter what the situation. When you have a choice, get off on the left so the drivetrain is out of the way as you push. If you need to carry the bike over your shoulder, always hoist it from the left side. Otherwise, you'll get smeared with chain lube and gouged by the chainrings.

If the course has a steep drop-off that you're uncomfortable riding, don't be too macho to dismount and run instead. Be smarter than the people who will end their race by crashing on sections that are too advanced for their skills.

Sitting

Stay in the saddle as much as possible. Early in the race, you'll be tempted to stand and jam out of turns, over short rollers, and across the tops of climbs. Sometimes, this is the right thing to do, but don't stand unnecessarily. Standing always uses more energy than sitting does.

In most races, I quickly reach a point where I'm too gassed to stand. That's why I usually do at least 90 percent of any race sitting down. I'm so close to my anaerobic threshold while sitting that standing pushes me right over. You'll be in the same situation when you're riding at race pace.

Attacking

If you're a great sprinter, you don't need to worry about dropping the guys you're with before the finish. But if you're more like me—not a particularly powerful rider—you'd better eliminate the opposition somewhere before the end. Good sprinters can smell the finish line, and the closer it gets, the deeper they'll dig to hang on. To get rid of them, you need to attack their weaknesses.

As a race wears on, you can tell where another rider struggles or makes mistakes. Maybe he's not really fast on flat ground. Maybe he tends to let up over the tops of climbs. Perhaps he fumbles on technical sections. In the last situation, for instance, you want to be ahead of him when entering singletrack. The harder you go, the more mistakes he's likely to make while trying to keep up. Similarly, take the lead on the final hill if he tends to give in as climbs end. The key is to reach these crucial sections first so you don't have to get past him in order to use your strategy. Otherwise, he could block you or the course may not be wide enough for a pass, handing the advantage back to him.

The same tactic can help you get rid of several riders at once. For example, suppose you're a good descender and you notice that one of the guys you're with has lousy downhill technique. You certainly want to attack past him going into a crucial descent. Then you can turn it on and lose him, maybe for good. With luck, he'll hold back everyone else in your group, giving you a gap that you can keep to the finish.

If the table is turned, do the opposite. Let's say that the guy you're trying to beat is a better climber. He's been gapping you on every hill. Coming into the race's crucial climb, you know that if he gets away, you won't see him again until the postrace barbecue. Hold him back by getting to the hill first. Delay his pass as long as possible. Then use your own strengths to pull him back and attack him before the finish.

My goal is to enter technical sections ahead of any riders I'm with. I don't want to risk being slowed down. If you follow this approach, you'll be able to maximize whatever technical riding abilities you have. If your speed happens to be slower than what the guys behind you could do, so much the better.

Although drafting isn't a major factor in most mountain bike races, pacing often comes into play. By pacing, I mean the tendency of a rider to key in on your speed and stick with you even though he may not be quite as strong. If you suspect that this is happening, attack to open a gap of 25 yards or so. All of a sudden, he'll slow down and settle into his own pace. Then you can back off and ride at the same level you had been, but without him in your hair. This is a useful tactic at any time during a race. The longer you let a guy stay with you, the harder it could be to lose him near the end, when his confidence has risen.

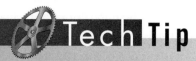

Tech Tip

Mechanical breakdowns are disastrous in races. All the preparation, time, and money that it takes to get to an event can be wasted in the instant when a part malfunctions. It's bound to happen sooner or later, but you shouldn't let it happen more than once to the same part.

Learn from the experiences of other riders. When I see a guy sitting beside the trail, I take a quick peek to check what happened. Did his chain break? Did his derailleur lose a jockey wheel? Did a pedal snap off? Did the fork blow?

If I hear after the race that a guy finished despite a problem, I track him down to discover what went wrong. By cataloging such failures, you can learn which brands may be unreliable or which are at risk in certain conditions.

Don't be the guinea pig for a company's product-development department. If you are going to try something new, do it in training before racing on it. Racing is the ultimate proving ground, which is why some of us are paid by companies to ride their products. Even so, we won't use something in competition until we prove to ourselves that it's effective and reliable.

Passing

Passing is a huge part of cross-country racing. On singletrack, the field must ride in a line, which lets gaps open between riders. If you don't quickly get past a slower guy, riders who are in front of him will be gaining ground that you may never get back.

Singletrack is often lined with no-passing zones—things you can't ride on, like rocks, trees, streams, hillsides, or ravines—so you need to watch for wider sections and make the most of them. When you're ready, yell "Track!" and announce the side that you want to pass on. Most of the time, this is all that it takes. The guy will move over a bit and you can surge by. Ideally, each of you will keep full momentum; that's what defines the perfect pass.

On the other hand, some people can make passing very tough. They may be obstinate, rude, or so focused that they don't pay attention to you. It may help to let a guy know if you're in a different racing class. He has nothing to gain by holding you back. Sometimes, it helps to set things up by announcing that you're back there and waiting for an opportunity. When you see it, say, "Now, on your left" (or right) and he will usually be more inclined to let you pass.

My tactic is to be polite. I never start out by yelling at someone, but I admit that sometimes I end up screaming. Different riders respond to different approaches. For instance, if I know the rider's name, it may work to say, "C'mon, Lenny, let's go. We can't let those guys get away." He may be inspired to pull us up to them. Or I say, "Let me close that gap for us." He's apt to move over immediately to let me by. Be tactful and use some psychology. Believe me, it works a lot better than, "You're slower than sludge, pal. Get out of my way!"

At other times, you have to be aggressive and rely on your riding abilities. Here's a good example from the Iron Horse Classic. I could see the leaders opening a gap on the guy in front of me. I yelled that I was going to pass on the right, but he wouldn't move over. Okay, plan B. We came to a fast section. I veered off the side of the trail and pulled even with him, but he still wouldn't slow down to let me get ahead. I was using a tremendous amount of energy to ride over bushes in the soft dirt. Finally, I had to slide back in behind him. I was gassed, right at my limit. I wasn't able to make another attempt for five minutes.

I finally got him in a turn—often the best place to pass on singletrack. You can count on centrifugal force to pull the rider to an outside line, opening the door for you. When he goes into the turn, dive through on his inside. This gives you a shorter distance to the exit, plus he'll tend to move over when he sees your wheel come though. Be aware of this tactic if the roles are reversed and you're trying to keep an opponent behind you. Block him from passing by taking a tight inside line through turns.

Sometimes, you find yourself in a back-and-forth passing duel. This can happen when you and the other guy have opposing strengths. Pro racer John Tomac and I have had many such battles because he is so great on downhills but I often climb better. I remember one national championship at Edgemont Ranch in Colorado when the two of us were duking it out. I passed him on the long climbs, then held him at bay on the descents by not moving over when he caught me. I made him wait to find sections that were wide enough. Then he dropped me, but I caught him again going up the next climb. Of course, he held his ground to keep me behind him for as long as possible. That's good racing.

On the final downhill, John opened his jets to get the biggest gap possible. He knew that his chance to win hinged on getting far enough ahead that I couldn't catch him on the climb to the finish. That's when he went flying into some tight turns and stacked it. When I arrived, he just happened to be blocking the trail with his bike. I couldn't pass, so we rode together into the last hill, where I got away for the victory. John had blown his downhill advantage by crashing, then we reached the uphill that favored me.

When the singletrack traverses a hill, always pass on the high side. Look for spots where you can ride up the slope. As soon as the other rider is aware of your front wheel, begin moving down. This forces him to steer to the downhill edge and let you back on the trail. Have enough speed and aggression to end his thoughts of challenging your pass. If you try to pass on the downhill side, the other rider can easily force you off the trail. You're putting him in command of the situation. When you come down from the uphill side, you're in charge.

I don't mean to suggest that you should pass in ways that could cause a crash and injuries. If there's a cliff along the trail, don't force someone to the edge or put yourself in a risky position. Singletrack presents an endless variety of situations. Wait for a few seconds for a safer place to pass.

Refueling

If a race lasts less than an hour, practically all of your energy can come from what's stored in your body, primarily the glycogen in your muscles and liver. You can get a few hundred extra calories on the course and stay hydrated by putting a sports drink in your bottles.

To maximize performance in races that are longer than an hour, you should definitely use a sports drink and perhaps energy gel. It's important to experiment with these products in training to find out how well you digest them during intense riding. I've tried various drinks over the years and I settled on those that contain both simple and complex carbohydrates. I find that they give a steadier supply of energy. I shy away from drinks that have a boatload of other ingredients. They seem to be better for marketing performance than for cycling performance.

I like powder drink mix because I can make my own fairly light solution of 100 to 125 calories in a 20-ounce bottle. To reach this level, I simply adjust the mixing directions as necessary. During a typical 2½-hour pro race, I try to drain one bottle every 30 to 40 minutes, depending on the heat and humidity. If it's cold, I make the solution a little stronger so I can get the same number of calories even though I drink less. (Try defizzed cola late in a long event. Dilute it about 50 percent with water. It's a fairly simple sugar source that also has some caffeine for a boost when energy is running low.)

In addition to sports drink, I suck down three packets of gel, one every half-hour or so starting 30 minutes into the race. One packet supplies about

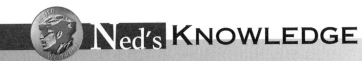

Here are some important do's and don'ts for cross-country racers.

Don't fudge in line. Sometimes, the field is so big and the singletrack starts so soon that there is a major logjam. Riders charge away from the line, then suddenly they're standing still again, impatiently waiting for the guys in front to move ahead on the singletrack. The temptation is very strong to walk or ride around the outside of the bottleneck to get back in the race. Don't do it. In fact, if other guys see you try this, they may not let you in line. I've seen shoving matches and even some punches.

Don't be overly courteous on singletrack. If you're in front of your competitors and bobble a section, there's no rule that says you have to pull over to let them pass. Hold your ground. Everyone makes bike-handling errors. Don't make a bigger mistake by giving up your place in the standings. Make them earn their way around you.

Move over if you're really messing up. When I'm blowing a section with four or five riders right behind me, sometimes they say something. Or maybe they don't, out of respect. But I know that they're there, and I know that I'm not riding well. In this case, I let them through—not the whole field, just until there's a gap that lets me jump back in. This usually works in my favor because I can relax and ride faster without the pressure of someone right on my wheel.

Yield to a mounted rider. Let's say you've gotten off to walk up a hill. Up from behind comes a guy who is still riding, making an effort to clean the climb. You don't have to stop and move aside, but show the guy some respect by walking outside the obvious line. You have a lot more choice in where to push your bike than he does in where to ride his. Show more sportsmanship by giving him an encouraging "Yeah!" as he churns past (especially if he's not in your competitive class).

Stop for someone who's hurt. This isn't necessary if there are spectators around, but when you're in the middle of nowhere and you find a guy down in a crash, you have a moral obligation to stop. Make sure he is conscious and breathing. If he's not in a life-threatening situation, tell him that you'll alert the next course marshal to send help. If in doubt, stay there. Tell the next passing rider to give the alert. No race is so important that you should leave a badly injured person alone in the woods.

Keep your cool. It's easy to get frustrated with other riders. I've passed guys who have dropped their bikes and started wrestling in the woods. Keep your temper, keep your focus, and keep your mouth shut. After all, if you're not able to control your emotions in a race, you won't be able to control your bike, either.

100 calories, so all told, I get at least 800 calories out on the course, plus I stay hydrated. Gel is much easier to get down than anything that you have to chew before swallowing. It makes no sense to attempt to eat solid food during a cross-country race. Besides the difficulty, it takes too long to digest and release the calories.

In hot weather, I carry one bottle of plain water in addition to my sports drink. I use it if my stomach goes south and can't handle any more sweet drink. Also, water works better for washing down gel. And sometimes, you need to rinse burning sweat out of your eyes—not something you'll ever try a second time (at least not intentionally) with a sports drink.

I don't use a backpack-style hydration system in pro races, because I can get a fresh bottle from my support team each time I pass through the hand-up area. If you don't have this luxury, consider one of the smaller-quantity systems that aren't too heavy or bulky. Combined with bottles on your bike, you can carry plenty of sports drink and water. The system's hose lets you drink anywhere on the course instead of waiting for smooth sections where you can reach for a bottle. Another advantage comes if you race or train on trails that are used by cattle or horses. Their stuff could contaminate your bottle tops as it flies up from the trail, with serious consequences for your digestive system.

Immediately after the race, you can do yourself lots of good by drinking more carbohydrates, along with some protein. Following long, hard exertions, your body is anxious to replenish glycogen, the main fuel for your muscles. It's easiest to do this with a commercial high-carb drink. Have a big bottle mixed and ready in your cooler. You'll recover faster and feel stronger the next day. Don't waste this opportunity by filling up on plain water.

Your first meal after a race should also be rich in carbohydrates and proteins. Proteins are important for rebuilding muscle cells damaged by strenuous riding. You need a nutritious meal so your body can refuel and repair.

Finishing

Get familiar with the finish area before the race begins. This is easy at an event that ends at the same place where it starts. For a point-to-point race, you may need to ask a race official for a description. What you're interested in is the amount of straightaway before the line, which determines the best tactic if you're finishing with other riders close by you.

Most cross-country courses aren't designed for the long, straight sprints typical of road events. In mountain biking, we tend to have a short finishing chute just past a sharp corner. In this case, the tactic is pretty simple. You need to be the first rider to the corner so you can take the fastest line through it. If you're in front on the short straight, there probably won't be enough distance for even a strong sprinter to get past you. It's similar on a course that has a smooth track flanked by thick grass or rough ground. If you're first into the track, other riders will have to swing out into the slow stuff to try to get by.

In a lap race, you have a chance to examine the finish each time around. Think about the best gear to be in. Think hard because gear selection is a huge factor when you're going head-to-head with other riders. You should be in a cog or two smaller than the one you're using to end laps, so you can finish fast. You'll have to live with your choice, because changing gears after a sprint begins can cost you just enough time to lose a place. Be aggressive and give it all you have. Push aside any doubts. Attitude is hugely important at the end of a race.

In an event with a longer finishing straight, drafting can play a role. As in road racing, look for a fast rider to get behind, then swing out and jump past the guy right at the line. Doing that is easier said than done after an hour or two of hard riding. And in most races, it never comes down to a sprinting contest. Blinding speed simply isn't essential for successful cross-country racing. Power is much more important. It's what separates you from your challengers out on the course. The more power you possess, the more solo finishes you'll have.

Cooling Down

For most people, the race ends the instant that they cross the finish line. They can't wait to jump off their bikes. But you can do a lot to alleviate post-race soreness and stiffness by staying in the saddle just 15 minutes longer. Stop at your car, wipe off, grab a bottle of sports drink to start the refueling process, then take a spin on a flat, smooth road or even around a large parking lot. Pedal easily until you've stopped sweating, your breathing is back to normal, and your legs feel more mellow.

Stretch a bit when you get back to your car, then get out of your dirty clothes. If you hang around in your riding shorts, you're asking for trouble. A damp and dirty liner is a breeding ground for bacteria and saddle sores. Clean your face, legs, arms, and crotch with the soap and water that you've brought for this purpose. If the air is the least bit cool, put on something that will keep your muscles warm. Finally, stay off your feet as much as possible, to keep your legs relaxed.

177

Evaluating

Not every race unfolds just like you want it to. In fact, most don't, which is why you keep racing and learning and racing again.

When I think about races that left me totally satisfied, a couple stand out: the 1985 and 1986 national championships. Those courses were pretty technical and hilly. I got into a groove. I felt mechanical, like my legs were just a couple of pistons. I was flying but not taxing my cardiovascular system to the max. I remember how relaxed I felt on the descents.

But some days, you don't win. In fact, you ride a lot worse than you should. This even happens to pros, and I'm no exception. Maybe you just can't reach your cardiovascular potential, or maybe you make a mistake that shakes your confidence and knocks you off your game. Often, a descent is involved. Something happens to give you a scare and make you tense. You can't relax, so you pull the brakes too much, which transmits more shock through the bike. This fatigues your arms. Now, your control deteriorates. You grab the brakes harder to cut speed for the turns. By the time you reach the bottom, you're riding in slow motion. The problem has escalated all the way down the hill.

When this happens, don't give up. Breathe deeply, relax the tension that you're feeling, and refocus. Sometimes, first laps go this way, then you get your focus back. By the last lap, you're grooving again and the race is a success after all. The key is not pressing to overcome mistakes. Just relax, slow down a bit, and mentally start over. Ignore what has happened so far and look forward to the riding that remains.

Bad stuff happens. If you can identify the cause of a bad performance, be sure to work on the problem until you conquer it. The wrong approach is to accept shortcomings. If I hear, "I'm not a good downhiller" or "I'm not a good climber," I know that the person is not really riding to his potential. Recognize your limitations but don't accept them. Fix them.

22 Training for Cross-Country

On-Bike Workouts
for the Road and Trail

In this chapter and the one that follows, I'll give you my recommendations about training for cross-country racing. During my 20-year career, I've learned a lot from personal experience, coaches, teammates, and the guys I've competed against. What I'm about to tell you, combined with the many bike-handling skills already covered, will explain what I do to develop the power, strength, and stamina necessary to race well in cross-country events.

In addition to these guidelines, you need a sharp sense of self-evaluation. This is what it takes to determine when to train hard and how much to rest—what I call the intensity/recovery ratio. It's critical because your body's ability to get stronger and fitter depends on cycles of tearing down and rebuilding. When you stress your muscles and cardiovascular system with hard riding or weight training, that's only half of the equation. Adequate rest must follow. Otherwise, you see only physical deterioration and loss of enthusiasm instead of a rebound to greater strength and fitness.

My approach to training is not as scientific as others'. One reason is that I didn't have a coach to learn from when I began racing. Instead, my system evolved through two decades of discovering what works and what doesn't. I rarely use a heart-rate monitor, and I've never followed a systematic plan that breaks up the year into strict quarterly, monthly, and weekly cycles, plus specific daily workouts. When I stand back and look at what I do, however, I realize it's actually a lower-tech version of the same thing. My intuitive approach is shared by other self-coached mountain bike racers, but I also know quite a few guys who prefer a more regimented system.

In order to coach myself well, I keep up-to-date with exercise research and training theories. I'll certainly add a new technique to my program as long as it doesn't restrict the flexibility that I need to keep training interesting. I just don't have much tolerance for rigid structure. I've been able to continue racing year after year by making training enjoyable as well as successful. The best proof to me that I'm doing it right is the fact that I still love to ride my bike, get fit, and go fast. This chapter will tell you how I do it. Then you can shape a program that fits your unique combination of age, talent, goals, time, climate, and terrain.

The Heart of the Matter

A rider needs to develop three aspects of fitness to become a strong mountain biker: aerobic endurance, anaerobic capacity, and the overall muscle strength that it takes to withstand the punishment of off-road riding. The last element results from a combination of weight training and riding on rough technical terrain (for more information on weight training, see chapter 23). Aerobic endurance and anaerobic capacity are improved by riding with a range of intensities that develop the cardiovascular system. The best way to do this (especially if you're new to training) is with guidance from a heart-rate monitor (HRM).

First rule: Be a bit flexible with the advice that follows. We're not machines. Many physical and emotional episodes in daily life can negatively affect individual stress levels and the ability to recover from the rigors of training. Don't discount the toll taken by such things as work, school, family relationships, insufficient sleep, illness, or even a missed meal. Cycling occurs in the context of a whole life, something that many enthusiastic riders seem to overlook.

An excellent source of detailed heart-rate workouts and in-depth training theory is *The Cyclist's Training Bible* by Joe Friel. This book is aimed at roadies, but the training programs and coaching advice will work for mountain bikers, too.

Begin by determining your lactate-threshold heart rate (LTHR). Lactate threshold (also called anaerobic threshold) is the point at which the debilitating by-product of hard exercise, namely lactic acid, floods your

Ned's KNOWLEDGE

My training advice is only loosely based on the numbers provided by a heart-rate monitor (HRM). Most coaches and some riders swear by digital readouts and the heart-rate zones that they define. I know that training by the numbers is important. However, my career started before the advent of reliable HRMs, so I never got into using one. Instead, I learned to use feedback from my legs and lungs.

To race well, you need a feel for how much energy any given effort is taking. That's the key to correct pacing. You could do this with a HRM, but I don't recommend using one in competition. It can be dangerously distracting when racing wheel-to-wheel and trying to negotiate technical terrain. Also, if your heart rate is higher than what you expect to see, your sense of exertion and fatigue may start matching what you do see, with negative consequences for your performance.

I believe that a rider's most reliable performance monitor is his gut feeling. For example, if I'm doing three five-minute hill intervals, I push myself to the level that I feel I can maintain for the duration, then hold it there. When my legs start burning, I'm where I need to be. If they begin getting the thickness that means lactic acid accumulation, I'm just over the edge and need to back off. Similarly, I want my breathing to be rapid but short of panting or hyperventilating. On shorter intervals, I may intentionally go beyond these points because that's what happens in racing. I lock in on the top of the hill and blow past my lactate threshold. I know I'm going anaerobic and can't keep up with my oxygen needs, but I can hold my speed and recover over the other side.

A HRM is a useful learning tool because it lets you correlate all this subjective feedback with actual heart rates, then train in the zones that they define. As time goes by, you can become very good at guessing what the monitor says based on the stress and fatigue you feel.

In a race, you must constantly self-monitor everything. How is your body reacting? For me, a full feeling in my legs is not a problem. I can back off slightly and let the lactic acid recede. But if I go beyond this point and feel tightness in my thighs and hamstrings, I know that my legs are in danger of not recovering no matter what I do. I then use lower gears to reduce the pressure. My objective is to ride just below the redline so I can get the most out of myself but still have some energy for the end of the last lap. Early in a race, I base my effort on how I'll feel in the next hour, not just in the next 5 to 10 minutes.

To race well, you must know yourself. Train your built-in monitor every time you ride.

muscles faster than it can be eliminated. LTHR is the highest heart rate that you can maintain for an extended period. In other words, it's your primary race pace. The purpose of training at your LTHR is to increase the amount of time your body can work at that intensity, allowing you to ride fast longer. When discussing training effort, it's a much more meaningful number than maximum heart rate. In fact, the most important thing about max heart rate is moving your LTHR closer to it, which indicates that your fitness is improving.

A good way to find your LTHR is by racing in a 10-mile road time trial. Be well-rested and feel fresh. Use a flat course that will let you maintain your absolute fastest speed throughout. If your HRM calculates average heart rate, that's ideal. If it doesn't, note the highest heart rate you see during the majority of the ride. To determine LTHR, I recommend Joe Friel's method of dividing this average heart rate by 1.05. For example, I time trial at a heart rate of 183 beats per minute (bpm), so my lactate threshold is 174 bpm. (*Note:* If you're riding the time trial in training and don't have the motivation of competition, divide by 1.01.) By the way, most people's LTHRs will be 15 to 18 beats below their maximum heart rates.

Now that you have your LTHR, you can easily calculate your heart-rate training zones. Friel identifies seven of them, but we can concentrate on these four as being most important for cross-country racers.

Zone 1: 65 to 81 percent of LTHR. At this range or below, you can actively recover, spinning through short rides to help loosen your muscles and flush out the by-products of hard training or racing.

Zone 2: 82 to 88 percent of LTHR. This produces aerobic endurance, so it's the right level for building a fitness base early in the season. It teaches your muscles to burn fat (not just carbohydrates) for fuel and prepares them for the greater stress and effort of interval training and racing.

Zone 3: 94 to 100 percent of LTHR. Training right at your lactate threshold maximizes your aerobic endurance. This is the predominant heart-rate range during racing.

Zone 4: 106 percent (or more) of LTHR. This takes an all-out effort that usually can be sustained for no longer than one minute. Training at this level boosts cardiovascular capacity and conditions you for the anaerobic efforts of fast starts, short steep climbs, and attacks to drop your competitors.

As you train in these various zones, focus on how your body feels in each one. Correlate heart rate to your breathing and the sensations in your muscles. This is essential to the learning process. The goal is to know your heart rate at any level of exertion without looking at your HRM. In cross-country racing, it's often risky to take your eyes off the course to check the numbers, and it's even difficult to see them clearly through the vibration.

Yearly Snapshot

My year-round program has one objective: to prepare me to race well in the most important events of the season. This is probably a goal that you share with me. Use my example to construct your own schedule, making adjustments based on when you want to have your strongest performances.

December through January: Build strength with weight training. Maintain cardiovascular fitness with cross-training and easy rides to keep a fluid pedal stroke.

February through March: Continue weight training while increasing time on the bike to build an aerobic base.

April through May: Reduce riding volume but increase intensity to prepare for early-season races.

June through July: Combine high-intensity training and racing to reach a fitness peak in the middle of this period. Then reduce intensity while maintaining volume to recover for a second buildup.

August through September: Increase intensity again to build toward a second peak for the big season-ending championships.

October through November: Reduce training. Race and ride for fun using residual fitness. Take time off from cycling and enjoy other sports.

On-bike training takes two forms: road and off-road. Although a mountain bike can be used for each, I recommend that you also have a road bike. When it comes to road training, it's simply the right tool for the job.

On-Road

There's one huge benefit of training on the road: You can get all of cycling's cardiovascular benefits without getting beaten up. The world's top cross-country racers do a lot of skinny-tire training because nonstop mountain biking is just too punishing. If you limit yourself to off-road training, you can't work out as much because you need more time for recovery.

Another plus is how much fun it is to ride a road bike. If you're used to spending all your time on a mountain bike, it's like trading in your baggy swim trunks for a Speedo. The smooth, nimble speed is a mental refreshment, and the dynamics of group riding add a new dimension to fitness. You pull hard in a paceline, jump to open a gap, sprint for city-limit signs, and

TRUE STORY

If you're interested in trying your hand at road racing, keep riding your mountain bike, too. Part of your preparation for road events can (and should) take place off-road. Mountain biking boosts your ability to handle skids, slippery roads, unexpected excursions off the pavement, and even riders who go down in front of you.

I remember the credit that Andy Hampsten gave to his mountain biking experience when he won the Giro d'Italia in 1988. Andy and I had occasionally ridden and raced off-road together in the old days, before he became a Europe-based pro roadie. In the Giro, a three-week stage race, Andy took the overall lead on a mountainous day struck by a freak snowstorm. He had to climb and descend a major pass in blizzard conditions on a snow-covered dirt road—on skinny tires yet. Not only didn't he crash but he also gained enough time to become the first North American to wear the leader's jersey.

When your tires are at risk of losing traction, remember Andy in that stage race and know when to brake. Braking hard in turns or during a skid will only put you on the ground. You can't have control unless your wheels are free to turn. This goes for any slippery situation on pavement or dirt. Once the tires stop sliding, steering and braking become more effective. Andy learned this on his mountain bike, so his instincts were right on his road bike.

constantly react to riders in close quarters. The skills gained on the road help you become a complete cyclist.

You can't get exactly the same position on a road bike as on your mountain bike, but it's important to come close. You want maximum carryover of conditioning while minimizing aches and strains. In particular, pay close attention to the saddle location relative to the bottom bracket. Strive for the identical height and fore/aft position on both bikes. To check the latter, drop a plumb line from the nose of the saddle and measure its distance from the center of the bottom bracket (crankset axle). Differences in seat tube angles, crankarm lengths, shoes, and pedal systems can complicate fore-aft accuracy. Be as precise as you can.

Interval training: A road bike is ideal for riding intervals, a type of workout in which you alternate periods of intense effort with periods of easy effort for recovery. One goal of this training is to raise your lactate threshold so you can ride longer at higher heart rates.

When you approach your lactate threshold, your breathing changes to panting and your leg muscles feel fiery and thick. Then you slow down and struggle to recover. This is why a high LTHR is key to racing success. The closer it is to your maximum heart rate, the faster you can ride. The best way to raise your LTHR is with zone-3 training efforts that repeatedly take you to the painful edge (or just past it). These hard efforts are interspersed with recovery intervals of easier riding. As you can see, this also simulates what happens in a race. Interval training pushes up your lactate threshold and lengthens the time that you can remain there.

An adequate warmup is essential for this training. I ride for at least 20 minutes and do a few short surges to elevate my heart rate and body temperature. Sometimes, I do extended time trial–like intervals, perhaps using a long, gradual climb that helps get my heart rate up. Or I actually compete in local club time trials for extended work in zones 3 and 4.

My favorite road workout is hill-climb intervals. They give me two benefits: LTHR training and muscle power. On pavement, I can concentrate on putting pressure on the pedals without concern for maintaining traction or avoiding obstacles. All of my energy goes into the effort. I focus on my breathing and how my legs feel.

I do hill-climb intervals on a steep-but-steady grade that takes about eight minutes to climb. I ride to the top, make a U-turn, recover by spinning on the descent and the flats, then go again. For variety, I change gears and tactics. For instance, sometimes I do the first seven minutes seated in

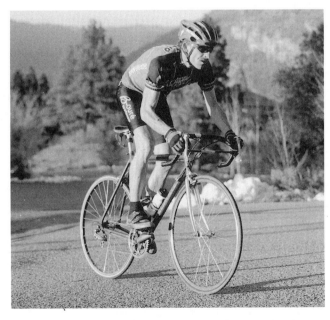

Training on a road bike lets you concentrate on your workout instead of on picking your way through obstacles. One of my favorite ways to use skinny tires is to do hill intervals, a very effective way to raise lactate threshold and improve power.

zone 3, then shift up and explode out of the saddle in zone 4 for the remainder. This simulates a long climb in a race where you attack at the top to gain position for the descent, then recover from the anaerobic effort. Or, I may attack the first half while standing, then sit and spin a smaller gear to the top. The position change makes it feel like I'm working two entirely different muscle groups. By starting in anaerobic zone 4 and then trying to recover as the climb continues, I simulate the common race situation of being buried in oxygen debt with a lot of hill left.

Watch your HRM during hill training and notice what happens when you change between sitting and standing. Most riders see a higher heart rate when they're out of their saddles, because it takes more energy to support their bodies. The trick is to minimize the increase with efficient technique, such as swaying the bike from side to side so body weight can help drive each pedal stroke.

Depending on the time of year and my fitness, I do from four to eight of these climbs during a workout. My rule of thumb for these or any intervals is to stop when I feel that I have just one more left in me. It's not good for the last effort to become ragged—that's how muscle and tendon injuries happen. Also, it's easier to recover from hard workouts if you don't totally overextend yourself. When you honestly doubt that you can maintain speed and form one more time up the hill, that's when you should turn around, congratulate yourself on a great workout, and enjoy an easy spin home.

Generally, I do hill-climb intervals once a week. My other hard workouts during each seven-day period consist of off-road intervals (discussed later in the chapter) and a weekend race or group ride.

Racing is actually the hardest workout of all, which brings up the question of recovery. Hard work without sufficient rest leads to overtraining and deteriorating performance. Typically, I do my interval training on Tuesdays and Thursdays so I have recovery time between workouts and before a weekend race. But let's say you rode a killer cross-country race on Sunday. Maybe you went out too fast, blew up, and finished with cramps and deep muscle fatigue. There's a good chance that you'll still be feeling hammered on Tuesday rather than recovered. Be honest with yourself and push back your interval training to Wednesday. Maybe that's the only hard workout you'll do that week if the next race is on Saturday. Be smart and be flexible. You'll get better if you're fresh for interval workouts and races. You'll get overtrained if you're not.

Group riding: The dynamics of group riding are unique to the road. Sure, when you go trail riding with your buddies, you tend to push each other on climbs and duel on downhills, and that's great. But for pure action, nothing beats riding with a fast pack of roadies. Drafting, attacking, chasing, sprinting—the result is like intervals but without any regimentation. This makes training much more interesting, and training actually seems easier because it's fun. As you pull hard in the paceline, try to escape, or try to close a gap, your heart rate is automatically redlining. Unlike specific interval training, there's no need to stare at a monitor and force yourself to make the number go higher. Spirited group riding will raise you to another level of fitness, and it teaches riding skills that you can't get on a mountain bike. The faster the group, the more you'll get out of it.

If you have the opportunity, take a ride like this once a week. It can substitute for interval training or even replace a weekend race. You'll see improvement in your top-end speed and ability to ride longer at your LTHR.

Endurance: If you need better stamina, zone-2 road rides of three to four hours will do the trick. On the other hand, off-road rides of that length will create much more fatigue because of all of the jolts and vibration. By adding one long, steady road ride to your weekly training schedule (Wednesday is favored by many riders), you can build muscle endurance and train your body to burn stored fat for energy.

Don't go overboard. Most cross-country races last less than two hours. This puts a premium on power and riding skill, not endurance. The hours it takes to do a very long distance ride and recover could be better spent developing strength, raising your LTHR, and working on bike handling. In the preseason, however, long road rides can be useful for building a base of aerobic conditioning and burning off weight gained during winter.

Recovery: Any strenuous training ride tears down a certain amount of muscle. When you ride hard on a rough trail, it gets worse—resistance coming into your legs through the pedals causes additional abuse. The result is intensifying fatigue late in the ride and cellular damage that increases muscle soreness and delays recovery.

What you need the next day is active recovery. Better than complete rest, an easy zone-1 ride will revive your stiff muscles through movement and increased circulation. But you won't get this gentle experience if you go off-road again (unless you have a dual-suspension bike and flat terrain). On a trail, there's always going to be more pounding and bike-handling effort. On pavement, you can relax. You don't even have to think about getting your butt off the saddle for rough sections.

The day after competing in a cross-country race, spin on your road bike for 60 to 90 minutes to aid recovery without taxing your energy system. Keep your heart rate in zone 1, and shift to a lower gear anytime you feel pressure on your legs.

Off-Road

There's a long list of road racers who've made very successful transitions to cross-country racing. Steve Tilford, Bob Roll, Steve Larsen, Jerome Chiotti, Juli Furtado, and Alison Sydor are names that come immediately to mind. I fit the description, too. Even superstar roadies like Greg LeMond and Lance Armstrong have given fat-tire racing a shot. Greg's career was winding down when he rode a few events for fun, and he even won Wisconsin's Chequamegon Classic.

Lance, on the other hand, was 26 and a top road pro when he jumped into a big U.S. cross-country race during a break from Europe in 1998. He led for more than a lap, but then the field overtook him. This showed that there's a lot more to successful mountain bike racing than awesome horsepower. "It was technically very difficult, with some crazy descents that were pretty scary," Lance said afterward. He'll vouch for the need to train on trails to prepare for the bike-handling challenges of cross-country racing. I'm sure that we haven't seen the last of Lance in fat-tire races.

Upper-body conditioning: Some riders need to train off-road to get extra work on certain skills, but there's a conditioning factor that benefits everyone. It's a sure bet that if you want the strength to race well on rough trails, you need to train hard on rough trails.

If you mainly ride your road bike and then jump into a cross-country race, you notice much more fatigue in your hands, arms, and shoulders. These muscles don't get conditioned well-enough on a road bike. Pete Penseyres learned this firsthand when he rode a long-distance mountain bike stage race in Costa Rica. Pete, an ultramarathon rider best known for his two victories in the Race Across America, had trouble sleeping during the off-road event because of frequent cramps in his arms. "I haven't used the brakes that much in more than 400,000 road miles," he explained. "The downhills were like nothing I was trained for. Mountain biking is sure different."

Off-road riding is a whole-body exercise. You need to ride trails often enough to keep your muscles accustomed to the demands. Include an occasional longer ride on technical terrain. Compared to endurance training on your road bike, this will develop more strength and stamina in your upper body. Don't overdo these rides. Recovery always takes longer than for a road ride of similar duration.

Interval training: To mix upper-body conditioning with some serious cardiovascular training, ride off-road intervals. These do a great job of simulating the demands of cross-country racing. My favorite rough workout is on Animas Mountain near my home in Durango, Colorado. There's a loop that includes a 25-minute climb followed by a 15-minute descent. I warm up on the ride to the base of the mountain, then do two laps. I start each one at a pace below my LTHR, then build to my zone-3 threshold for the final 10 minutes to the top. It's a great workout because the trail is rocky and twisty as well as steep.

This is an awfully long "on" period for an interval, so I don't recommend that you do an exact copy. Begin with four or five minutes of intense effort and work your way up from there. If you don't have a suitable loop, just ride the same trail up and down. Don't use one where the climbing is too technical for your ability, or you'll be picking your way around obstacles instead of ascending with enough effort to stay in zone 3.

On the other hand, the tougher the descent, the better for training. Riding off Animas is like going through a minefield. Hard tire pressure is a necessity. You ricochet from one rock pile to the next, learning to pick lines and unweight over things that can't be avoided. This works your hands and forearms especially hard. In this situation, you need a firm grip on the handlebar but not a death grip. Your arms need to be loose enough to absorb shock. To prevent your forearms from pumping up and seizing, you need to find spots where you can relax your grip on the brake levers every few seconds.

On the other side of Durango is what we call the Telegraph ascent, which loops into the Anasazi descent. Here, I do a different type of interval training. These trails are much smoother than on Animas Mountain but the descent is very tight, with at least a dozen switchbacks. I do three zone-4 efforts of a minute apiece going up, alternating with five-minute zone-2 recovery intervals. Then, I really force the speed all the way down. I get the benefit of hard anaerobic climbing for power development, plus high-quality downhill practice that explores the limits of cornering traction, which is the key to getting better on descents. You have to push yourself right to the edge and risk an occasional fall as you practice the downhill techniques discussed in chapter 14.

This training works even better when I ride with friends and we battle each other up and down. It's the ideal way to do off-road intervals—incorporated into rides that also enhance bike-handling skills. If you're riding alone, however, stay just to the inside of the envelope on descents. A hard crash could be life threatening if there's no one to help you.

Other types of interval training (the varieties are many) can be dictated by what the terrain throws at you. For instance, make up your mind to jam every hill on a rolling trail. After you've warmed up, start flooring it. Practice finishing each hill by pushing hard over the top and into the descent. Ride easy to recover between these zone-3 and -4 efforts. This workout will improve your leg strength, cardiovascular power, and sense of how hard you can go in an actual race.

Wall banging: I don't know of any paved climb that can put the intense pressure on my legs that I feel on Chapman Hill. This little ski area in Durango is so steep that I don't have to push myself to reach zone 4. It happens automatically on every trip to the top. A typical workout consists of four to six repeats up this 500-yard-long wall. It takes everything I have. The stress on my knees and hips is almost supernatural. This training gives me a definite advantage in the Iron Horse Classic, which starts with this same climb.

Find your own Chapman Hill—the most vertical piece of real estate in your area—then train on it once every two to three weeks. That's plenty. Be well-rested beforehand, then take a recovery day afterward. You'll get mental as well as physical benefits. When a wall looms up in a race, you'll know that it can't stop you.

Group riding: When I'm training off-road, I prefer to do it alone or maybe with just one or two other guys. That way, I can focus on exactly what I want to accomplish. Going with a group is fun sometimes (especially in winter, when it's cold and you're just getting some saddle time), but if you're always with others, you won't improve as quickly. This is particularly true when you're working on skills or doing intervals.

I know that some people hate riding alone. If that's you, it's still important to do at least one solo ride each week to practice bike-handling drills and riding in specific zones. Focus, and you won't miss the company.

Recovery: There are days when I need to recover but I still feel like riding in the woods. It's times like these when a dual-suspension bike is ideal. I notice a lot less soreness after any hard ride on my dualie, and this same plushness also makes an easy trail ride possible. I granny gear almost every climb and simply enjoy the afternoon. If I'm with friends, we chat the whole way. Rule of thumb: If you're having trouble keeping up a conversation during a recovery ride, it's a sure sign that you're going too hard.

When others join you for a ride like this (or for any ride, for that matter), have a clear understanding of the pace you're going to keep. Any group ride is at risk of turning competitive. Go with riders of a like mind, and limit the number. When you're out with 10 others, it seems like every five minutes someone is flatting, dropping something, jamming a chain, or crashing. You end up just waiting around for half of the time. Small groups work better.

And remember, there's nothing wrong with a day off. Let's say you've been training hard and are due for some rest. You also have a late meeting at work, a list of errands to run, and a bike that could use some maintenance. It's fine to schedule a day for all these other demands and let it double for resting your legs. Lots of people rest for one or two days each week. Personally, I like to get some exercise every day, so I rest by taking one-hour zone-1 spins, or I might go swimming or jogging. If I'm more sore than tired, a short, easy ride always makes me feel better than doing nothing at all.

What about a longer break? When you're training enthusiastically but your progress stalls or even reverses, it's likely that you're doing too much. Most people think the opposite, that they need to work harder, and so they're in the downward spiral of overtraining. Instead, think about taking a week off even in the heart of the season. The history of bike racing has many examples of riders who came back with great results after being forced to stop training. I remember when Don Myrah broke his collarbone in mid-season, took some time off, then had the best performance of his career to win the NORBA world championship at Mammoth, California. Then there was top pro Daryl Price, who developed a skin infection after a crash, missed time while on antibiotics, then crushed us at a NORBA national in Big Bear, California.

Such injuries give riders a physical and mental break that they would never take voluntarily. I think the fact that subsequent performances are so strong indicates that most people train and race too much. It's easy for enthusiastic riders to become compulsive. Do your best to be objective about how you're feeling on the bike. If you're literally going nowhere fast, a short vacation could renew your energy and attitude. Staying completely away from the bike usually works better than a week of recovery rides. They tend not to be easy enough, plus there's hardly any mental relief.

Sample Week

Putting it all together, here's what a typical week during the season may look like for a cross-country racer. Maybe this fits your schedule very well, or maybe it won't work for you without adjustments. Design your own mix

Ned's KNOWLEDGE

It's hard to beat the benefits of an hour with a skilled massage therapist. The relief that it gives to sore, fatigued muscles following hard training or racing is phenomenal. Even a routine once-a-week massage makes a difference that your body will appreciate.

For pro racers, massage is a necessity. For other riders, it falls more into the category of a luxury, and not an inexpensive one, at that. Fortunately, there's self-massage. It isn't nearly as relaxing as having someone work on you, but it is effective, especially for your legs.

I do a short routine almost every day, usually right after training, when my muscles are warm and full of blood. It consists of slow stroking movements for my calves, quadriceps, and hamstrings. As I push the blood back into circulation, I feel for little knots and tight places that often develop during hard rides. By working them out immediately, they don't become real injuries.

This routine takes only five minutes per leg. Later in the evening when I'm stretching in front of the TV or listening to music, I work on sore spots again.

of hard work and recovery. Remember that progress comes faster if you go really hard on the hard days and really easy on the easy days. Training at nearly the same pace all the time will make you fitter, but not fit for racing.

Monday: Zone-1 recovery ride following the weekend's hard training or racing

Tuesday: Zone-3 road intervals

Wednesday: Day off, or long steady zone-2 ride for endurance

Thursday: Zone-4 off-road intervals

Friday: Day off, or zone-1 recovery ride with some skill drills

Saturday: Race, or short zone-1 or -2 ride with two brief hard efforts if race is on Sunday

Sunday: Race or zone-3 or -4 group training; zone-1 recovery road ride if race or hard training was on Saturday

Winter Rides

In winter, you need to build a fitness base for the upcoming training and racing seasons. In colder climates, this typically means plenty of road miles.

The windchill created by riding around at 17 or 18 mph can make it tough. Even on a calm, sunny day, temperatures around 30°F will feel like they're in the single digits.

In these conditions, I switch to my mountain bike even for pavement riding. The fat tires increase rolling resistance and lower my speed, making it seem less cold. I'm also better equipped to deal with potholes, patches of snow or ice, and the gritty stuff that maintenance crews spread on the roads.

Stay warm by dressing with neoprene shoecovers, and a waterproof, breathable jacket, layered over a jersey that will wick moisture away from your skin. In sloppy conditions, you may need tights that have a waterproof shell on the front of the leg. Add a hat and balaclava to protect your face and a pair of "lobster" mittens for your hands, and you're ready for battle. Check chapter 23 for more on winter training.

23 Winter Training

Workouts That Boost Performance and Enthusiasm for a New Season

In mountain bike paradise, we'd ride endless singletrack all year-round in perfect weather. But here on Earth (and especially in my hometown of Durango, Colorado), there is winter. It gets dark before dinner and numbingly cold in northern regions. Trails get buried by snow. Even road riding is difficult because of frigid windchills and treacherous patches of ice. Yeah, from December to March, it's tough being a bike rider.

I have a simple philosophy: Don't fight it. Winter is nature's way of making us take a break from routine riding, and that's good. Even paradise could get boring without some variety. My approach in the off-season is to reduce saddle time. But even where it stays warm through the winter, you should voluntarily cut back on cycling.

The challenge is to turn the off-season into a positive period. Without riding, it's easy to feel deprived in winter. Get rid of that feeling by following an alternative program that's fun and satisfying and that helps you enter spring ready to ride even better than the previous year. Done right, this training is as refreshing for your head as it is productive for your body.

A smart winter program also builds reserves. Imagine that you have a full tank of gas when you start the season. Gradually, through the year, you will use most of it. I'm not talking only about physical energy. I also mean the motivation to continue riding and racing. If you empty your tank completely, you'll be in the ditch, unable to continue. Winter is where you refill your tank with enough gas to last until the next off-season fill-up.

Bikers Beware

There's no doubt about the benefits of winter training, but before we go further, I must warn you: It also can ruin your season. I've seen coaches prescribe intensive programs, and I've seen riders follow them enthusiastically. The guys go into the spring absolutely flying. Then in July, they're dead—physically and mentally burned out. There's nothing left for the heart of the season. It's interesting to see who wins the Cactus Cup that's held early each spring in Arizona. He's usually not the rider who wins the important races in July and August.

I knew an expert-level racer with lots of talent who trained enthusiastically in winter. He watched his diet, spent time in the weight room, and doggedly rode every day, right through the gnarly Durango weather. He did intervals in February and was unbeatable in April. Two months later, he actually retired from the sport.

He's not the only one this has happened to. I see riders of all skill levels drain their tanks. The only solution is to stop riding long enough to recover energy and rebuild desire. But just try to convince anyone to take a week off.

My winter approach is different. I train with weights to get overall body conditioning. I want to strengthen the muscles that mountain biking misses as well as the muscles that it uses. I do other sports for fun, variety, and their aerobic benefits. I take some casual rides to keep me accustomed to pedaling. Sometimes, I spin on the resistance trainer when an extended period of bad weather stops me from riding outside.

The result is that I stay fit in winter, but not cycling fit. All rides are easy, and any intensity comes from the sports that I do for cross-training. I don't force myself to follow a rigid program, and I make sure to never get mentally tired. Using this approach, I feel refreshed and hungry for on-bike training when spring begins. In April and May, I want to have good performances but not top performances. Spring training and racing should be stepping stones toward great rides in mid to late summer, when the most important events take place.

When you're near top form early, you see only small increments in improvement as the summer progresses. The guys you were beating in May could start beating you in June. This can be very discouraging. You feel like you're fading when actually it's they who are coming on strong. So you train harder, become overtrained, and really regress. It's much better for your enthusiasm and motivation if you can see significant progress all through the season. I'm a come-from-behind racer, and I guess you could say I'm a come-from-behind trainer, too. I decide when I want to be in top form, then plan backward.

Complementary Sports

In winter, I like to cross-train with running, cross-country skiing, snowshoeing, and swimming. All of these sports, combined with some cycling, help maintain my cardiovascular system. Skiing and swimming have the added benefit of strengthening my upper body. Snowshoeing, with its emphasis on the lower back, quadriceps, and glutes, is probably the most complementary to cycling. It can be a real power workout on days when you're feeling energetic.

These sports can actually open new competitive opportunities. Now that I'm no longer racing full-time as a pro cyclist, I've begun competing in the new multisport event called X-Terra. This is like a traditional triathlon except that the running and cycling take place off-road. I've been doing well because so few competitors have mountain biking backgrounds. They lose time to me on technical climbs and descents. I need this advantage because I give most of them a big lead in the water. In the run, I rely on my background in track and cross-country. I can't run a 4:25 mile anymore like I did in high school, but I can hold my own, especially in the hills.

Except when competing, my main objective in these other sports is to enjoy the exercise. I'm not doing them specifically to improve my cycling, but of course they do help by keeping me fit through the winter. I like the way they work different muscles and refresh my body.

Running is particularly important for mountain bike racers because we sometimes need to run for short sections in an event. Use winter to introduce running to your program, starting with uphill jogs. The leg action is similar to pedaling, so it doesn't stress your muscles in unaccustomed ways like the long strides of regular running do. Walk, don't run, down the hills, or the pounding will have you hobbling the next day. Uphill running is the most common type that you'll do in off-road racing. It's a great cardiovascular workout, too. Just be patient when you start. Once your legs have adapted, you'll be free to run in any terrain. Always go easy on descents to reduce stress on your knees.

Participate in any other sport that you enjoy. Soccer can be a good workout, and it's great for balance and coordination. The same goes for basketball. I also like sports such as table tennis that improve hand-to-eye coordination, which is a key skill in mountain biking. You encounter something with your eyes, then you react to it with your hands. The martial arts are good for this, too, and they improve flexibility.

Swimming is helpful because it teaches breath control. You expel all of your air underwater, then refill your lungs during the brief moment when your head is turned to the surface. To improve in swimming, you need to relax, and that's a good lesson for mountain biking. You can't have tense muscles and swim or ride your best. When you remember to relax your neck and shoulders while climbing, for instance, your whole body benefits. Swimming can give you a fine workout in 30 minutes, if you're pressed for time. It's good exercise for your back and shoulders while being very gentle to your body overall. Give it a try even if you're a hacker in the water. After all, poor form makes it that much easier to get your heart rate up.

Cycling Indoors and Out

In December and January, I ride about three days a week. I say about because I don't force it. For instance, let's say I've planned a two-hour ride, but it's snowing or 20°F with a hard wind blowing. A very unpleasant ride is waiting for me. I could do it, but the intensity would be so low that I wouldn't miss much by bundling up and skiing or running instead. Always remember that you want to enter spring hungry for cycling. This won't happen if you force yourself to get on the bike in winter.

Winter is an excellent time to improve technical mountain biking skills without feeling any pressure to do a hard workout. I spend lots of time doing what I call crash-avoidance drills, working on balancing, trackstands, nose wheelies, unweighting, tight turns, and clipping in and out of the pedals. Even when it's dark or you're snowed in, these skills can be practiced in the basement or garage.

There's another cycling alternative, of course. You can clamp your bike into a resistance trainer and ride indoors. I can't say I'm a big advocate—I'd much rather be doing anything outside—but I realize it's the only way that many people can fit some pedaling into their winter weekdays. Even if you're not forced indoors by darkness, riding inside does have some advantages. For example, let's say spring is approaching and you'll soon be increasing your on-bike training. Suddenly, there's a spell of bad weather. Instead of missing rides or suffering in miserable conditions, you can use the trainer to stay on schedule.

Many people (myself included) find riding indoors mentally difficult. The first pedal stroke is usually the hardest—climbing on the darn thing and getting started. It helps to listen to fast-paced music; watch a video; keep changing your gears, cadence, and effort; and limit workouts to an hour. Don't just sit there and grind at a steady pace. Nothing makes a clock run slower than that does, and it won't do nearly as much for your fitness as interval-type workouts, where you vary your speed and intensity throughout the workout.

If you must use a trainer for your main aerobic activity in winter, don't overdo it. An hour every other day is as much as I recommend. Remember the importance of mental refreshment at this time of year. Use alternate days for weight training, and do your best to include other aerobic activities.

Rollers are another indoor option. I actually like them better than a resistance trainer because they make you balance the bike. This gives you something else to think about. In addition, rollers help develop a smooth, round pedal stroke that carries over to outside riding.

I've spent some time on a CompuTrainer, too. This high-tech resistance trainer is probably the most effective device for riders who are either confined to indoor cycling for long periods or who actually prefer it. Among other benefits, a CompuTrainer simulates outdoor riding by automatically changing pedal resistance in synch with the terrain of courses displayed on your TV screen through a Nintendo hookup. You can get a very good workout by racing against the internal computer or your own previous performance. Another feature, called Spin Scan, shows you how much pressure you're applying to the pedals all the way around each stroke. This helps you identify and correct poor technique or imbalances. A CompuTrainer makes indoor cycling about as interesting and effective as it can be.

Benefits of Weight Training

Although I occasionally trained with weights during much of my cycling career, I discovered that I wasn't doing it well enough. Like many hard lessons, this one arrived in the form of a racing experience.

After our classic battle at the 1990 world championship in Durango, Swiss racer Thomas Frischknecht and I were at it again in 1991 in Luca,

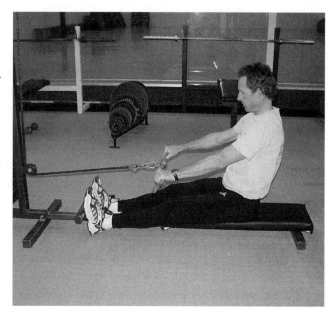

Here's one of my favorite cycling-specific weight exercises. These seated rows develop upper-body strength for lofting the front wheel and climbing. Space your grip the same as you do on a handlebar. You can also use a bar with vertical handholds to simulate gripping bar-ends.

Italy. Only this time, we were fighting for the silver medal. Pro racer John Tomac, who has never climbed better than he did this day, was long gone and about to win his first world championship.

In Durango, when Thomas dismounted to run up the steep hill, I stayed on my bike and beat him. This time, in Luca, Thomas turned the tables on me. We both had to run through a long section that torrential downpours had turned into a quagmire. Thomas is a strong, powerful guy who excels in cyclocross as well as in mountain biking. I did my best, but it was no contest. Our bikes weighed a ton because of all the mud covering them. Thomas had the strength to hoist his awkward 35-pound piece of gooey machinery and run like a deer. I felt more like a 98-pound weakling struggling in quicksand. As I watched him disappear, it became clear how important extra strength can be in mountain biking. When all else is equal, the guy with the stronger body has the advantage.

Balance and Flexibility

Aside from strength, there's another big benefit to weight training: muscle balance. The problem with riding a bike is that it builds some muscles very well while ignoring others. Weight training turns cyclists into whole athletes again. For instance, pushing on the pedals is great for developing your quadriceps, on the fronts of your thighs, but it does almost nothing for your hamstrings, on the backs of your thighs. Leg curls improve the balance and reduce your risk of hamstring tightness and injury.

In a similar way, cycling stresses your lower back much more than it stresses your stomach, so it's important to do crunches to strengthen your abdominal muscles. An uncorrected imbalance can result in lower-back pain and poor posture.

Flexibility is another benefit. Traditional weight lifting emphasizes fewer repetitions with heavy resistance, which can shorten muscles. My approach of many repetitions with moderate resistance through the full range of motion tends to stretch my muscles and keep them supple and elastic. When I'm riding, this helps me move all over the bike for better control, and it reduces the risk of muscle pulls during falls. In this sense, weight training helps prevent crash damage.

Toned muscles also protect you in a way that's often overlooked. When muscles are larger and denser, they put more tissue between your bones and whatever you're landing on. A bruised muscle heals a lot faster than a broken bone. Think about football players. They don't bulk up in the weight room just to be stronger. They know that muscles provide pro-

Ned's KNOWLEDGE

Because I travel a lot, it's hard to maintain my weight-training schedule. Perhaps you're in the same situation, or maybe you occasionally get stuck at home or work on a day when you're scheduled to be at the gym. My physical therapist turned me on to a neat little product that has saved my workout many times.

It's called the Xertube, from SPRI Products. It's simply a length of elastic tubing that comes in five thicknesses for different resistance levels. Prices are under $10. A strap for fastening one end to a door is a little extra. An Xertube lets you do several exercises for your legs as well as for your upper body. Add some crunches, pushups, lunges, or step-ups to get a workout that you can feel good about. Call (800) 222-7774 to order this product.

tection in a contact sport. For cyclists, the question is how do we get this benefit without unnecessary bulk. High-rep, low-weight exercises are the answer.

The Program

My strength-training program includes about 20 different exercises. This is a lot, but I go to a well-equipped health club, so I make the most of the equipment.

You don't need to do so many. Once you get past the basic lifts, there's a lot of redundancy in the muscle groups that are strengthened by weight training. Depending on the equipment available, design a routine that gives some work to every part of your body. If you're unsure how to do that, there are many books on the subject. Even better, get advice from a professional instructor at the gym where you work out. The professional also can coach you on proper lifting form, which is crucial for maximizing results while minimizing your risk of injury.

A good upper-body routine for mountain bikers includes crunches, back extensions, bench presses, military presses, bent rows, upright rows, lateral pulldowns, dumbbell flies, triceps extensions, and biceps curls. For the legs, include hamstring curls, short-arc leg extensions, calf raises, and leg presses (or squats if you have a rack and spotter).

I also like to use the abductor/adductor machine to strengthen my groin muscles and expand my legs' range of motion. This exercise and some of the others won't necessarily help you ride your bike better, but they develop lateral strength that can counteract the twisting forces of a crash.

If you have access to the equipment, seated rows are a great cycling-specific exercise for the upper body. I do them two ways. First, I position my hands and arms like I'm holding handlebar grips and pull straight back to my chest. Then, I turn my hands to the position they're in when gripping bar-ends. I make sure my hands are spaced the same way that they are on my bike's handlebar. These rows develop strength for climbing and for lofting the front wheel.

Workout Schedule

Hit the weight room two or three times a week, always with at least one recovery day between workouts. To warm up, I pedal a stationary bike for about 15 minutes to break a sweat, then stretch for 15 minutes. I use the circuit-training technique of moving directly from station to station without rest between. I alternate upper- and lower-body exercises so half of my body is recovering while the other half is working. This brisk pace is intended to make efficient use of time, not to turn weight training into an aerobic workout. My goal is to be in and out in 90 minutes. Most cyclists are beyond the fitness level where hustling through a circuit workout will give them much cardiovascular benefit.

In my experience, cyclists get a good balance of strength and safety by using moderate resistance that allows two sets of 12 to 15 repetitions for each exercise. I do one set of each exercise, then go through again. This works muscles throughout my body with about 30 total reps of each exercise. I finish with 15 more minutes of stretching to keep my muscles loose and reduce soreness.

This high-rep approach strengthens muscles without adding much bulk. Strength is good, but extra body weight isn't desirable for hilly cross-country racing. On the other hand, power-oriented riders such as downhillers, trackies, and road sprinters don't have to worry about a few more pounds. To maximize strength, they bulk up with greater resistance and fewer reps.

There are two other reasons to use less weight and more reps. One is injury prevention. I've learned firsthand how easy it is to get hurt at the health club. If you don't lift year-round, you run a high risk of muscle strains and pulls early in a weight program. Your shoulders and hamstrings are particularly vulnerable. Lighter weights reduce the danger.

The second benefit is psychological. It's a mental as well as a physical strain to lift heavy weights. Because you know that each exercise is going to be hard and even painful, it isn't long before workouts become distasteful. Quitting usually isn't far behind.

Remember, our sport is mountain biking, not power lifting. I've learned to start each winter program like a 98-pound weakling rather than like Arnold Schwarzenegger. You need to swallow your pride in the weight room. When that 100-pound woman gets off the machine, reduce the weight before you take over. Machismo will only get you injured. Err on the side of using a bit less weight than you can handle, rather than too much.

I admit that this isn't the way to get absolute maximum strength benefits, but in order for weight training to help you, it has to be done consistently. Many riders fizzle out because of the stress, soreness, and time requirements of an overly ambitious program. Be realistic. A schedule of just 10 different exercises twice a week will be beneficial if you maintain it throughout the winter.

Keep doing 12 to 15 reps of all upper-body exercises and, as your training progresses, increase the weight only enough to make yourself keep pushing pretty hard as you do the last two reps. Stop one rep short of absolute maximum. Always pushing to the limit in each exercise raises your risk of injury if your form breaks down. You're using too much weight if you can't reach 12 reps in the second set or if the effort is causing bad technique.

It's different for leg exercises. After your muscles have adapted, begin adding weight and decreasing reps as a way to build power and strength. Don't go overboard, though. The weight should never be so much that you can't do at least 10 reps. The one leg exercise that I really emphasize is hamstring curls. Because pedaling develops your hamstrings much less than it develops your quads, your hamstrings are more susceptible to injury if you don't remedy the imbalance. Once you can do 15 curls, add weight and build toward 15 again. Keep this up throughout the winter.

As spring gets closer, I reduce or eliminate redundant upper-body exercises, especially those that aren't cycling specific. Something has to give when riding increases, because there's only so much time and energy for training. I spend what's left of my weight sessions on exercises for my legs, such as step-ups, lunges, hamstring curls, and leg presses. I also continue to do crunches and back extensions. They're essential for your body's core support system—the balance between your lower-back and abdominal muscles.

Do this maintenance program once a week throughout the racing season. You need it to retain the strength and flexibility that you build in winter. During some weeks of hard training or racing, you may not have the time or energy to hit the weights, and that's okay. Just don't stop weight workouts completely.

Back on the Bike

After enjoying other sports in December and January, start to rebuild your cycling base. A good way is by doing social rides with your buddies. Don't go hard, and don't worry about going long if you live in a cold climate.

It's tough to do three-hour rides in freezing temperatures. Your legs will feel like wood. Consider using your mountain bike until the air gets warmer. It's slower than a road bike, so windchill is reduced.

This is also the time to increase what I call your body's support mechanism. As you start to ride more, there's more stress and, thus, more of a chance that you'll get sick. To fight this, keep your immune system strong with enough sleep, good nutrition, and plenty of fluids. And if you start to come down with something, back off. More than once, I've tried to train through a cold and turned it into a nasty sinus infection. Now, I always back off. The same goes for a tight muscle or sore tendon. Reduce riding and treat it with ice and massage so it won't get worse. It's a juggling act. Although you're trying to train more, you need to combat all of the little things that go wrong.

By the end of February, I ride the road or trails five or six days a week. March is usually my biggest training month in terms of time on the bike. I seek overall conditioning and stamina, so I put in 15 to 18 hours per week, mostly in heart-rate zone 2 (for more information about heart-rate zones, see chapter 22). This is a lot—probably 25 to 50 percent more hours than recreational racers need to do. Sometimes, the pace gets fast if I'm riding with a group, but I don't do specific interval training in March. It would be different if there were races I was trying to perform well at in April, but my schedule is aimed at trying to be competitive in late May.

April's training is more specific. The quantity is down a bit from March, but the intensity is higher. In early April, I incorporate zone-3 intervals during the week with races or fast club rides on the weekend. The competitions sharpen my bike-handling skills and reveal my conditioning weaknesses so I know what to focus on in training. By the second half of April, I add some zone-4 intervals to the mix. This combination of base miles, intervals, and strength work prepares me to begin serious racing and continue building fitness. Group rides and races are a great way to do speed work because it is easier to get motivated. When you're chasing guys or they are bearing down on you, you just go. When you are doing intervals alone while staring at your heart monitor, it requires more mental energy to push yourself to the limit.

In May, I start traveling to races. This reduces my training time, so I back off from endurance and emphasize power and speed. In June and beyond, I circle the dates of championship races and train specifically to do well in them. If I'm riding up to my potential in July, August, and September, my season has been a success.

Winding Down

Autumn is a beautiful time to be on a mountain bike, so I make the most of it. All the major championships are over, though there are still a few races and festivals. Festivals are great because they take you back to the reasons that mountain biking is so much fun. I look forward to riding at them. By October, I've had it with the physical and mental stresses of hard training, so I rely on my residual fitness and the events themselves to keep me performing respectably. The only intervals that I'm interested in are the ones between where I'm staying and the restaurants.

I also begin the transition into cross-training. I do some trail running to enjoy the fact that snow has yet to cover the ground. If I feel like taking a total break, I take it. A couple of weeks off in November or early December brings closure to the season and makes me really want to get started again. By training this way, I know that I'll keep my enthusiasm for years to come. I hope you will, too.

Glossary

Aerobic: An intensity of exercise that allows the body's need for oxygen to be continually met. This intensity can be sustained for long periods.

Anaerobic: An intensity of exercise above that at which the body's need for oxygen can be continually met. This intensity can be sustained only briefly.

Anaerobic threshold: *See* Lactate threshold (LT).

Apex: The sharpest part of a turn, where the transition from entering to exiting takes place.

Attack position: A well-balanced riding posture in which the elbows and knees are bent and flexible, the butt is just above the saddle, the torso is low, and the head is up. This position is used to float over rough ground, prepare for unweighting maneuvers, and so on.

Balaclava: A thin hood that covers the head and neck with an opening for the face. It's worn under the helmet to prevent heat loss in cold or wet conditions.

Bead: In a tire, the edge along each inner circumference that fits into the rim.

Beginner: The NORBA category for novice recreational racers. A rider must advance to the sport category after placing in the top five in five beginner races.

Berm: A small embankment along the edge of a trail, often occurring in turns.

BMX: Bicycle motocross. It refers both to the sport and to the bicycle, which has 20-inch wheels and a single speed.

Bonk: To run out of energy, usually because the rider has failed to eat or drink enough.

BPM: Abbreviation for "beats per minute" in reference to heart rate.

Bunny hop: A technique in which both wheels leave the ground to ride over obstacles such as rocks or logs.

Cadence: The number of times during one minute that a foot completes a pedal stroke. Also called pedal rpm.

Cardiovascular: Pertaining to the heart, lungs, and blood vessels.

Catch air: What happens when both wheels of a mountain bike leave the ground, usually because of a rise or dip in the trail.

Chainring: A sprocket on the crankset. Mountain bikes have three: the big, middle, and small (granny).

Chainsuck: When the chain sticks to the chainring teeth during a down-shift and gets drawn up and jammed between the small chainring and the frame.

Circuit training: A weight-training technique in which you move rapidly from exercise to exercise with no rest.

Clean: To ride a tough section without putting a foot on the ground to prevent yourself from falling over.

Clydesdale: A large rider. At some cross-country races, there is a Clydesdale class for riders who weigh more than 200 pounds.

Cog: A sprocket on the rear wheel's cassette or freewheel.

Contact patch: The section of a tire that is in contact with the ground.

Criterium: A road or off-road race in which competitors ride numerous laps around a short course.

Cross-country: The traditional and most popular type of mountain bike race. Most courses mix fire roads (where you can pass or be passed) with singletrack (where passing is difficult). Races may be point-to-point, one long loop, or two or more laps of a shorter loop.

Cross-training: Participating in several sports for mental refreshment and physical conditioning, especially during cycling's off-season.

Cyclocross: An off-road event in which the course has obstacles that force riders to dismount and run with their bikes.

Dab: To put a foot on the ground to prevent yourself from falling over.

Damping: Determines the rate of compression and rebound in a front or rear suspension. On most suspensions, damping is adjustable, letting you set the shock so that it returns to its original position in time for the next bump but doesn't recoil so fast that it makes the bike bounce.

Doubletrack: Two parallel trails formed by the wheel ruts of off-road vehicles. Also called a Jeep trail.

Downhill: A race held at a ski area. The fastest rider from top to bottom wins. Competitors wear protective clothes and pads ("body armor") and usually ride special dual-suspension bikes designed for maximum shock absorption.

Downshift: To shift to a lower gear, for example, to a larger cog or smaller chainring.

Draft: The slipstream created by a moving rider. Another rider close behind can keep the same pace while using about 20 percent less energy.

Drift: When inertia or centrifugal force pulls the bike off-line, often in a turn. Also called wheel drift.

Dualie: A bike with front and rear suspension. Short for "dual suspension."

Dual slalom: As in skiing, riders race downhill between gates on parallel courses. Unlike in a downhill race, in which the clock determines the winner, dual slalom is head-to-head elimination. Riders continue advancing until they lose.

Dual suspension: *See* Dualie.

Elastomer: A compressible, rubberlike material used to absorb shock in some suspension systems.

Endo: To crash by going over the bike's handlebar. Short for "end over end."

Expert: The NORBA category between sport and semi-pro. It's for riders who have developed advanced racing skill, strength, and stamina. Riders can remain expert for as long as they wish.

Fire road: A dirt or gravel road in the backcountry that is wide enough to allow access by emergency vehicles.

Glutes: The gluteal muscles of the buttocks. They are the key to pedaling power.

Glycogen: A fuel derived as glucose (sugar) from carbohydrates and stored in the muscles and liver. It's the primary energy source for high-intensity riding. Reserves are normally depleted after about 2½ hours of riding.

Granny gear: The lowest gear ratio, combining the small chainring with the largest cassette cog. It's mainly used for very steep climbs.

Granny ring: The smallest of the three chainrings.

Gyroscopic effect: The tendency of a revolving wheel to remain vertical. Called gyro for short.

Hamstrings: The muscles on the back of the thighs, which are not developed well by cycling.

Hardtail: A mountain bike with no rear suspension.

International Mountain Bicycling Association (IMBA): An organization dedicated to protecting and expanding trail access for mountain bikers. For information, write to IMBA, P.O. Box 7578, Boulder, CO 80306; or visit the Web site at www.imba.com.

Interval training: A type of workout in which periods of intense effort are alternated with periods of easier effort for recovery.

Lactate threshold (LT): The exertion level at which the body can no longer produce energy aerobically, resulting in the buildup of lactic acid. This is marked by muscle fatigue, pain, and shallow, rapid breathing. The heart rate at which this occurs is termed lactate threshold heart rate (LTHR). Also called anaerobic threshold.

Lactate threshold heart rate (LTHR): The heart rate at which the body can no longer produce energy aerobically.

Lactic acid: A substance formed during anaerobic metabolism, when there is incomplete breakdown of glucose. It rapidly produces muscle fatigue and pain.

LT: *See* Lactate threshold.

LTHR: *See* Lactate threshold heart rate.

NORBA (National Off-Road Bicycle Association): The division of USA Cycling that governs mountain bike racing. For information, write to NORBA, One Olympic Plaza, Colorado Springs, CO 80909; or visit the Web site at www.usacycling.org.

NORBA National: While NORBA sanctions hundreds of races each year, only a handful are part of its national championship series. Top finishers earn points that determine the season's overall winners.

Nose wheelie: A technique in which you elevate the rear wheel and ride on the front wheel only. Compare Wheelie.

Observed trials: A slow-speed event in which the objective is to ride a difficult, obstacle-filled course without putting a foot on the ground to prevent yourself from falling over. The winner is the rider who puts a foot down least often. Also called trials.

Off-camber: Turns in which the ground slopes toward the outside, making it harder to keep traction as speed increases.

Pedal rpm: *See* Cadence.

Pinch flat: An internal tire puncture caused by the tube being squeezed against the rim. It results from riding into an object too hard and makes two small holes. Also called a snakebite.

Plow: When the front wheel digs into a soft surface instead of responding to steering inputs, taking the bike off-line.

Preload: The adjustable spring tension in a suspension fork or rear suspension. It determines how far the suspension compresses under body weight and how much travel remains to absorb impacts.

Presta valve: The narrow European-style valve found on some inner tubes. A small metal cap on its end must be unscrewed before air can enter or exit.

Pro: NORBA's top racing category. Most professional racers are sponsored and travel the world to compete in major events.

Psi: Abbreviation for "pounds per square inch." The unit of measure for tire inflation and for air pressure in some suspensions.

Pushing: Pedaling with a relatively slow cadence using larger gears.

Quadriceps: The muscle group on the fronts of the thighs, which is well-developed by cycling.

Ratchet: To pedal back and forth in partial strokes. This allows a rider to pass obstacles that would cause a pedal to hit if it were to reach the bottom of a normal stroke.

Reach: The combined length of a bike's top tube and stem, which determines the rider's distance to the handlebar.

Rollers: A stationary training device consisting of three or four long cyclinders connected by belts. Both bike wheels roll on these cylinders so that balancing is much like it is when riding outdoors. Also, the term used to describe a series of short hills.

Schrader valve: An inner tube valve identical to those found on car tires. A tiny plunger in the center of its opening must be depressed for air to enter or exit.

Semi-pro: The NORBA category between expert and pro. It serves as a stepping stone for riders who aspire to race professionally as well as a way for pro teams to identify new talent.

Singletrack: A trail so narrow that two cyclists can't easily ride side by side, which makes passing difficult or impossible.

Snakebite: *See* Pinch flat.

Speedwork: A general term for intervals and other high-velocity training, such as time trials and practice races.

Spinning: Pedaling with a relatively fast cadence using small to moderate gears.

Sport: The NORBA category between beginner and expert. It's usually the largest field at any race. After finishing in the top five in five races, a sport rider must advance to expert.

Sprocket: General term for a cog or chainring.

Switchback: A turn sharper than 90 degrees. Switchbacks are found mainly on hills that are too steep to be ascended (or descended) using a direct path.

Technical trail: Singletrack filled with obstacles such as rocks, roots, logs, sharp turns, and steep grades, which put a premium on riding skills.

Track: The word to yell when you want a rider you're catching to move over so you can pass.

Trackstand: A skill where a rider comes to a full stop without putting a foot down. On a technical trail, a trackstand lets you pause to decide what to do next, and it may save you from toppling over if you suddenly come to an unexpected halt.

Travel: The maximum distance that a suspension fork or rear suspension can compress.

Traverse: To reduce the steepness of a hill by riding up in zigzag fashion. Also refers to a trail that cuts along the side of a slope.

Trials: *See* Observed trials.

Unweighting: Using a combination of body movement and position to momentarily lighten the amount of your body weight borne by the wheels of the bike. It's integral to techniques such as wheelies, bunny hops, and jumps.

Upshift: To shift to a higher gear, for example, to a smaller cog or larger chainring.

Wash out: When one or both wheels lose traction and slide toward the outside of a turn, taking the rider off course and perhaps causing a crash.

Wheel drift: *See* Drift.

Wheelie: A technique in which you elevate the front wheel and ride on the rear wheel only. Compare Nose wheelie.

Acknowledgments

Special thanks to Fred Matheny, Pete Penseyres, Geoff Drake, and Tim Blumenthal for their editorial assistance. Also to Christine Engleman for her faultless transcription of many hours of taped conversations between Ned and Ed.

Index

Boldface page references indicate illustrations. Underscored references indicate boxed text.

U

About the Authors

Ned Overend has won more elite cross-country races than anyone in the sport's history. Among his victories are a world championship, six national championships, and numerous World Cup events. In 1990, he was inducted into the Mountain Bike Hall of Fame. In 1998, at age 43 with his pro cycling career winding down, he opened a new chapter by winning the off-road X-Terra Triathlon Championship. Ned lives in prime mountain biking country in Durango, Colorado, with his wife and two children.

Ed Pavelka has written or compiled 18 books about cycling. His most recent work is *Bicycling Magazine's Complete Book of Road Cycling Skills*, also published by Rodale Press. He served as editor of *Bicycling* magazine from 1985 to 1997 and as editor of *VeloNews*, the journal of bicycling racing, for eight years before that. Now an independent writer, he works from his home in southeastern Pennsylvania. Ed rides in ultramarathon cycling events and passed 200,000 lifetime miles in 1999.